ETHICAL ISSUES IN RURAL HEALTH CARE

Edited by

CRAIG M. KLUGMAN
and
PAMELA M. DALINIS

The Johns Hopkins University Press
Baltimore

Johns Hopkins Paperback edition, 2013
9 8 7 6 5 4 3 2 1

The Johns Hopkins University Press
2715 North Charles Street
Baltimore, Maryland 21218-4363
www.press.jhu.edu

*The Library of Congress has cataloged the hardcover edition of this book
as follows:*

Ethical issues in rural health care / edited by Craig M. Klugman and
Pamela M. Dalinis.
   p. ; cm.
  Includes bibliographical references and index.
  ISBN-13: 978-0-8018-9045-1 (hardcover : alk. paper)
  ISBN-10: 0-8018-9045-4 (hardcover : alk. paper)
  1. Rural health services—Moral and ethical aspects—United States.
I. Klugman, Craig M., 1969– II. Dalinis, Pamela M., 1951–
  [DNLM: 1. Rural Health Services—ethics—United States. 2. Cultural
Diversity—United States. 3. Health Services Accessibility—ethics—
United States. 4. Healthcare Disparities—ethics—United States.
5. Medically Underserved Area—United States. 6. Rural Health—United
States. WA 390 E84 2008]
  RA771.5.E84 2008
  174′.957—dc22   2008015421

A catalog record for this book is available from the British Library.

ISBN-13: 978-1-4214-0955-9
ISBN-10: 1-4214-0955-0

*Special discounts are available for bulk purchases of this book. For
more information, please contact Special Sales at 410-516-6936 or
specialsales@press.jhu.edu.*

The Johns Hopkins University Press uses environmentally friendly book
materials, including recycled text paper that is composed of at least 30
percent postconsumer waste, whenever possible.

ETHICAL ISSUES IN RURAL HEALTH CARE

To those who provide health care in rural settings

CONTENTS

CONTRIBUTORS

Jamie Anderson, M.S., M.A., is the director of the Division of Interdisciplinary Medicine at the University of Nevada School of Medicine. She coordinates the advanced clinical experience in rural health care.

Martha Beard-Duncan, M.A., J.D., is an attorney based in Austin, Texas. Most recently, she has been working for Texas Rio Grande Legal Aid's Hurricane Relief Project. She was editor in chief of the *Houston Journal of Health Law and Policy* in 2004–2005.

Louis Borgenicht, M.D., is a practicing pediatrician in Salt Lake City, Utah. For two years he served in the U.S. Public Health Service on Wind River Indian Reservation in Wyoming.

Frank Chessa, Ph.D., is an assistant professor in the Department of Philosophy and Religion at Bates College, in Lewiston, Maine. He is also the director of clinical ethics at Maine Medical Center in Portland and vice president of the Maine Bioethics Network.

Ann Freeman Cook, Ph.D., is an associate professor in the Department of Psychology at the University of Montana-Missoula and is director of the National Rural Bioethics Project.

Pamela M. Dalinis, M.A., B.S.N., R.N., is Director of Education at Midwest Palliative and Hospice CareCenter in Glenview, Illinois. She is also a clinical bioethicist and ethics consultant at Elmhurst Memorial Hospital in Elmhurst, Illinois.

Marion Danis, M.D., is the head of the Section on Ethics and Health Policy in the Department of Clinical Bioethics at the National Institutes of Health, where she is also chief of the Clinical Bioethics Consultation Service. She is on the medical staff at the National Naval Medical Center.

Charles E. Gessert, M.D., M.P.H., is senior research scientist at St. Mary's / Duluth Clinical Health System and a clinical assistant professor of the University of Minnesota School of Medicine, in Duluth.

Dan Goodkind, Ph.D., has been a practicing psychologist since 1997 in Vernal, Utah, 170 miles from Salt Lake City. He is the director and owner of the Ashley Family Clinic in Vernal.

Helena Hoas, Ph.D., is an associate professor in the Department of Psychology at the University of Montana–Missoula and research director for the National Rural Bioethics Project.

Craig M. Klugman, Ph.D., is an associate professor in the Department of Medicine and Assistant Director for Ethics Education at the Center for Medical Humanities & Ethics at the University of Texas Health Science Center at San Antonio.

Julien S. Murphy, Ph.D., is director of the Bioethics Project and professor of philosophy at the University of Southern Maine. She is also president of the Maine Bioethics Network.

William A. Nelson, Ph.D., is the director of the Rural Ethics Initiatives and an associate professor of community and family medicine and psychiatry at the Dartmouth Medical School in Hanover, New Hampshire.

Denise Niemira, M.D., is a family practitioner at the Women's and Children's Health Center, Inc., in Newport, Vermont.

Elwood L. Schmidt, M.D., is a semiretired general practice physician who worked for 50 years in rural areas of Arizona, New Mexico, Nevada, and Texas. He still practices 10 hours a week in rural Lovelock, Nevada.

Elizabeth A. Thomas, R.N.C., Ph.D., M.P.H., is an assistant professor at the Texas Tech Health Sciences Center School of Nursing in Lubbock.

William J. Winslade, Ph.D., J.D., is the James Wade Rockwell Professor of Philosophy in Medicine at the Institute for the Medical Humanities, University of Texas Medical Branch, Galveston, and Distinguished Visiting Professor of Law and associate director for graduate programs at the Health Law and Policy Institute at the University of Houston Law Center.

PREFACE

Bioethics has had four areas of focus: theoretical, clinical, policy, and cultural (Callahan 1995). This volume brings together philosophers, lawyers, physicians, nurses, and researchers writing about rural ethics in each of the four areas. Interviews with rural practitioners are interspersed with chapters about research studies, theoretical papers, and discussions of rural challenges.

The chapters cover a range of rural areas across the United States. Gessert, Borgenicht, and Goodkind focus mainly on the West in their discussions of rural culture and medical practice. Schmidt discusses health practice, and Thomas writes about embedded structural violence in the Southwest. Cook and Hoas present research studies conducted in the Northern Plains. Nelson, Niemira, and Chessa and Murphy offer perspectives from New England. Winslade and Beard-Duncan talk about rurality in Texas. Anderson and Klugman survey rural medical training across the United States as well as in Canada and Australia.

The first part of the book looks at the differences between rural and urban in terms of defining rurality as well as ethical and health care challenges. Charles E. Gessert's chapter explores the differences in culture between rural and urban and how they affect views on end-of-life care for elderly people. William A. Nelson then offers a theoretical and clinical overview of the characteristics of rurality and discusses a range of ethical issues, such as conflicts, limited resources, challenges, dual roles for health care providers, and ethics committees. Nelson suggests that practitioners in rural health and scholars in bioethics need to pay more attention to rural bioethics. Ann Freeman Cook and Helena Hoas discuss theoretical and clinical findings from many studies conducted by their National Rural Bioethics Project. Their chapter examines how rural practitioners do not categorize various issues as ethical in nature. Marion Danis offers a regulatory and policy perspective on the limited resources available to rural health care practitioners and shows how various philosophical frameworks can help provide an understanding and a change in resource allocation.

The second part of the book offers personal clinical narratives by health care providers who have spent some part of their professional lives providing health care in rural settings. These three care providers share their experiences, challenges, and insights about working in varied rural locations across the West and Southwest. Their stories provide a perspective and understanding for people who have not worked in rural settings, and they also add a voice of practice experience. Elwood L. Schmidt recounts the challenges and ethical issues he faced as a primary care provider in rural Arizona, Nevada, Texas, and New Mexico over a 50-year career, including 11 years in an isolated town of 4,000 where he was the only doctor. Louis Borgenicht served as a pediatrician for two years on the Wind River Indian Reservation in Wyoming. Dan Goodkind is a practicing psychologist who talks about providing mental health services and running a mental health clinic in rural Utah.

The third section of the book deals with and proposes solutions to specific ethical challenges to rural health care providers and residents. Denise Niemira, a family practice physician in Vermont, writes about clinical issues, such as providing quality care and the rural physician's role, from being a community resource to maintaining professional competence. Frank Chessa and Julien S. Murphy pick up on clinical and theoretical themes from earlier chapters on ethics committees and support networks in rural areas. Their experience with the Maine Bioethics Network has given them perspective on how rural hospitals and health care providers can come together to provide ethics services and interests. Elizabeth A. Thomas offers a theoretical and policy discussion of entrenched structural violence in the lives of rural women on public assistance. William J. Winslade and Martha Beard-Duncan offer a policy perspective on aging in rural areas through their research and work in Texas. Jamie Anderson and Craig M. Klugman discuss how medical schools can provide clinical and policy support to practicing rural physicians as well as encourage medical students to experience rural practice and to consider working in those regions.

This book initiates a necessary collaborative conversation on the ethical issues and concerns facing rural health care providers. The chapters, although diverse, identify only some of the issues in rural bioethics. By presenting the causes of these issues and suggesting possible solutions, we hope that local and state policies may be implemented, leading to improved health care in rural regions.

The editors would like to thank the Nevada Center for Ethics and Health Policy for its unending efforts to improve health care in Nevada and in the nation. Without the support of Noel Tiano, Barbara Thornton, Betty Dodson, Peggy McGraw, Lisa Almada, Ginger Fenwick, Lizzie Romero, Trish White, and Alan Froman, this book would not have been possible. We also thank them for organizing the 2004 Rural Bioethics Symposium at Lake Tahoe, which became the seed for this book. The symposium was made possible by a Last Acts Grant from the Robert Wood Johnson Foundation.

We also thank our long list of tireless anonymous reviewers, who made key suggestions to improve each chapter.

Our thanks also go out to Thecla Ree for editing this volume and making sure that we did not get our dashes and hyphens confused.

Last, we thank our incredible writers, who wrote from their professional and scholarly experiences to make sure that this volume would be able to tell the story of rural need and rural triumph in relation to bioethics.

ETHICAL ISSUES IN RURAL HEALTH CARE

Introduction

CRAIG M. KLUGMAN, PH.D.

PAMELA M. DALINIS, M.A., B.S.N., R.N.

Before the notion of "rural medicine" evolved, medical and nursing practitioners assumed that taking care of rural residents was no different from caring for urban dwellers (Long and Weinert 1989). In the past, health officials believed that the main challenge of providing health care to rural residents was that the number of rural physicians was declining. The answer was to build health centers, and physicians would be attracted to practice in rural areas (Starr 1982). Experience has shown, however, that rural health practitioners have challenges beyond limited physical resources. The geography, the rural patient population, and ethical dilemmas are often distinct in scope and type from those of the urban practitioner. Unfortunately, bioethics has offered a limited literature or discussion of these challenges, instead focusing on individual patient care in technological settings (Klugman 2005).

Film and popular literary romance has depicted the rural practitioner as a noble hero bringing urban sophistication to a backward and often neglected community. In the film *Doc Hollywood* (1991), an educated urban physician brings modern medical practice and technology to a small town. While attempting to convert the local physician to his ways, he learns from the town residents poignant life lessons about how to better treat patients.

A. J. Cronin's 1937 novel, *The Citadel,* tells a different story. Andrew Manson, a young medical school graduate, accepts a position in a small, Welsh mining town. Andrew's impressions are far from positive. His description could refer to most small rural towns: "This strange town, primitive and isolated, entombed by the mountains, with no places of amusement, not even a cinema, nothing but its grim mine, its quarries and ore works, its string of chapels and bleak rows of houses, a queer and silently contained community" (Cronin 1937, p. 32).

Having come from a cosmopolitan medical center, Andrew is appalled by his working conditions and even more upset that practicing in such a small town may stigmatize him. With the distinction of "rural doctor" on his resume, he may be excluded from the excitement of cutting-edge medicine practiced in an urban research center. Andrew leaves the small town as quickly as possible to practice and perform research in London.

As shown in these fictional accounts, the experience of going to a rural area to provide health care has its challenges. The chapters in this volume show that the ethical issues and conditions of a rural health care provider are not the same as those in the urban setting. The contributors shed light on the unique ethical situations in which rural health care is practiced and suggest innovative, local responses.

How Is *Rural* Defined?

Unfortunately, no single definition of *rural* exists or is commonly used. As Nelson (chap. 2) points out, writers in the *Journal of Rural Health* used 26 different definitions over a two-year period (Johnson-Webb, Baer, and Gesler 1997). The United Nations (2007) does not define the term because such definitions differ widely by culture and country. Instead, the United Nations (2007) uses a notion of localities and population density within each "distinct population cluster." The U.S. government has three separate definitions of *rural*. The U.S. Census Bureau defines *rural* as all people who live outside of urbanized areas (UAs). An urbanized area is a dense population center that includes an urban core (which may or may not be a city) and surrounding developed territory. The area population must exceed 50,000 with a core population density of 1,000 people per square mile. Adjoining territory must have at least 500 persons per square mile to be included in the UA (U.S. Census Bureau 1995). The 2000 census defines as *rural* any territory, population, and housing units located outside of urbanized areas (>50,000 residents) or urban clusters (2,500–49,999 residents) (U.S. Census Bureau 2002a). According to the census definition, 59.1 million people (21% of the population) live in rural areas (U.S. Census Bureau 2002b).

The Office of Management and Budget uses the notion of metropolitan statistical areas (MSAs). Each MSA must include a city with 50,000 or more residents and a surrounding metropolitan area of at least 100,000 people (although in New England only 75,000 are needed). Thus, an MSA includes a central city as well as the city's county and any surrounding counties that add to the metropolitan population (Office of Budget and Management 2000). All non-MSA area is considered rural. As of 2000, according to this standard, 19,886,915 people, or 7.9 percent of the U.S. population, lived in rural areas (U.S. Census Bureau 2003).

The U.S. Department of Agriculture's Economic Research Service (USDA ERS) defines *rural* as an area that "comprises open country and settlements with fewer than 2,500 residents" (U.S. Department of Agriculture Economic Research Service 2003). They code counties based on their level of urbanization or proximity to metropolitan areas according to a scale from 0 to 9 (U.S. Department of Agriculture Economic Research Service 2004). By the USDA ERS definition, just over 17 percent (49.9 million) of the U.S. population lives in rural areas (U.S. Department of Agriculture Economic Research Service 2003).

In addition to the rural designation, areas may be known as frontier. The term *frontier* indicates those areas with fewer than seven people per square mile (Zelarney and Ciarlo 2000). For example, Alaska is a frontier state with a density of 1.1 people per square mile (U.S. Census Bureau 2002c).

Further confusing the notion of defining rurality is that the government definitions so far discussed are based on human population. Another way of looking at rurality is by land use. Is the land used for heavy urban development? Is it primarily agricultural? Is it primarily open space? How far is the land from the nearest concentrated area of development? When looking at a land-based definition of rural, one should realize that more than 94.6 percent of U.S. land is designated rural open space (O'Toole 2003). Thus, by the U.S. Census Bureau definition, approximately one-fifth of the population lives spread out over nearly 94 percent of all land in the United States.

No matter which definition one chooses, the essence of rurality is small populations spread over vast distances. Each of the authors in this volume spends some space defining *rurality*. Their individual experiences and research have drawn on these different definitions. Thus, because of the lack of a single accepted meaning for the term, the authors may not be consistent in their use of *rural*. Also, someone writing about rurality in New

England is talking about different distances from cities and population densities than someone writing about rural Utah or Nevada.

Trends in Rural Health Care and Populations

In most literature on rural health and rural life, writers assume that rural people are a homogeneous group with a static or shrinking population. Such a perception is highly inaccurate. The number of nonmetropolitan residents increased 2.2 percent from 2000 to 2005, with the greatest growth in rural areas that border urban centers (U.S. Department of Agriculture Economic Research Service 2007a). Rural areas also have a larger proportion of seniors (over 65) than the rest of the nation. Fifteen percent of rural residents are senior, versus 12 percent nationally (U.S. Department of Agriculture Economic Research Service 2007b). The existing rural population is growing older, and there has been a migration of seniors choosing to retire to rural areas, a topic that Gessert discusses in chapter 1 (U.S. Department of Agriculture Economic Research Service 2007b; Frey 1995; Rogers and Raymer 2001).

Rural communities are also culturally, ethnically, racially, and linguistically diverse. While ethnic minority populations have always called rural areas home, their percentage of the total rural population is increasing. According to the USDA ERS, 18 percent of rural populations are nonwhite (U.S. Department of Agriculture 2007c). Since 1980, the rural Hispanic population has doubled nationwide (Kandel and Cromartie 2004). In this volume, Danis (chap. 4), Winslade and Beard-Duncan (chap. 11) and Borgenicht (chap. 6) deal substantively with issues of diversity in rural life.

The way that health care is being delivered to rural residents is beginning a technological transformation. Over the past 30 years, the number of rural hospitals has decreased, meaning fewer hospital beds and less tertiary care medicine available for residents of those regions (Ricketts and Heaphy 2000). One response to this need has been the development of telemedicine programs. "Telemedicine refers to the use of electronic communication technologies to provide clinical care" (National Rural Health Association 1998). Health care providers in urban, tertiary care centers can advise, educate, and help treat patients who live in rural areas through the Internet, interactive video, videoconferencing, e-mail, electronic databases, and electronic records (Hassol et al. 1997). Between 2002 and 2007, the U.S. Department of Agriculture funded the more than 2,200 rural health care centers to develop telemedicine infrastructure (2007).

Health in Rural Areas

Rural residents report having poorer health and more physical limitations in performing activities of personal care and home management than their urban counterparts (U.S. Department of Agriculture Economic Research Service 2006). The large distances and small populations make accessing care challenging. Besides geography, another challenge can be found in the health problems experienced by rural dwellers.

The World Health Organization defined health as "a state of complete physical, mental and social well-being and not merely the absence of disease or infirmity" (World Health Organization 1948). This notion of health is expansive, taking into account social opportunities in addition to physical and mental states. In contrast, Long and Weinert determined that in rural areas, the notion of health is quite different and is defined as "the ability to work, to be productive, to do usual tasks" (1989, 120). As long as people can perform their necessary work chores for the day, no matter how many aches, pains, or infirmities they may feel, rural individuals will classify themselves as "healthy." Health means hardiness. The rural resident's self-identification with the concept of hardiness translates to being less likely to admit to health problems and seek assistance. Admitting pain or weakness may lead to dependence on others. Rural residents pride themselves on their hardiness, tending to be self-reliant, rejecting outside help such as urban doctors and government programs, and choosing instead to take care of each other (Bigbee 1991; Long and Weinert 1989; Neimoller, Ide, and Nichols 2000). The rural resident's trait of hardiness may result in not acknowledging disease in its earliest stages because usually one's work must be affected before a health issue is noticed. As a result, rural residents, when first seeking medical attention, can be sicker than their urban counterparts. Researchers find that the overall health of those living in rural areas tends to be lower than that of people in urban areas (Adams et al. 2001; Gillanders and Buss 1993).

People living in rural areas are more likely to have limited finances, to lack health insurance, to rely on Medicare at younger ages, and to have higher levels of psychological distress than people living in urban areas (National Center for Health Statistics 2004; Packham and Griswold 2007).

Mental health issues may not be acknowledged at all, and rural residents may not self-identify a need for mental health services even if urban researchers discern a need (Roberts, Battaglia, and Epstein 1999; Roberts et al. 1999; chap. 7).

Rural residents feel more connected to the land, their community, and their dwelling (Cooper 2006), causing reluctance to leave when they do encounter serious health problems. Thus, they are also more likely to want control over their deaths. Jared Diamond, in his book *Collapse,* interviews John Cook, a Montanan fishing guide:

> I often think about how I would want to die. My own father recently died a slow death of lung disease. He lost control over his own life, and his last year was painful. I don't want to die that way. It may seem cold-blooded, but here is my fantasy of how I would die if I had my choice . . . I would go trout-fishing every day as long as I was physically in condition to do it. When I became no longer capable of fishing, I would get hold of a large supply of morphine and go off a long way into the woods. I would pick some remote place where nobody would ever find my body, and from which I could enjoy an especially beautiful view. I'd lie down facing that view and take my morphine. That would be the best way to die: dying in the way that I chose, with the last sight I see being a view of Montana as I want to remember it. (Diamond 2005, 72–73)

John Cook's idea of health is being able to fish. When that's gone, he wants to die his own way, gazing out at the land that he loved. John describes a way of death that many rural residents prefer. Nationally, the rate of suicide is higher in rural areas than in urban ones (Eberhardt et al. 2001; National Center for Health Statistics 2004; Singh and Siahpush 2002). Ethnically, the highest rates are among Native Americans, followed by non-Hispanic whites. Rates for all other groups are about half of the two previously mentioned (National Center for Health Statistics 2004). For example, Nevada is classified as 87 percent publicly managed land with rural or frontier designations, with 10.7 percent of the population living in these rural and frontier regions (Packham and Griswold 2007). This state also has one of the highest suicide rates in the nation. The 2004 Nevada suicide rate was 18.2 per 100,000 versus 10.7 per 100,000 nationally. Nevada counties designated as rural or frontier led the suicide rate at 27.4 per 100,000 compared to 16.7 per 100,000 for the two main urban counties (Packham and Griswold 2007). Furthermore, the largest percentage of suicides in rural areas is among the elderly population (over 65 years of age) (DeJan and Yang 2005).

The Rural Health Practice Environment

The daily practice environment for the rural clinician is different from an urban trained medical professional's. Despite that 21 percent of the U.S. population lives in rural areas, only 11 percent of physicians practice in those same areas (U.S. Department of Health and Human Services 1996). Rural medical practices usually have fewer patients than urban practices, but the patients are spread over a much wider geographic area. The rural physician works longer hours and has more patient visits (American Medical Association 1996). More rural physicians are general practitioners than their urban counterparts (American Medical Association 1996), and they make less money (Frenzen 1996). As the chapters in this book demonstrate, rural practitioners often feel a strong sense of isolation from their peers and from the cutting edge of medical science.

The rural setting can be a shock to one who has not experienced it. The clinic itself often lacks many of the resources an urban-trained physician may expect. Instead of having separate facilities or units for different departments, the outpatient and inpatient clinics may double as the office, research lab, and cafeteria. In a report to the New York County Medical Society, state health commissioner Hermann Biggs described the isolation, lack of access to diagnostic technology, and lack of access to specialists: "Just think for a moment what it would mean . . . if you were cut off absolutely from all kinds of laboratory and x-ray service. If you were cut off from all association with your colleagues, from all assistance from specialists, and you were left to practice everything—every specialty in surgery, medicine, gynecology, obstetrics and everything else. Now that is exactly what the practice of medicine is in the rural districts of the State" (Starr 1982, 195).

Biggs's concerns are similar to those expressed by today's rural practitioners. However, Biggs gave this address in 1920. Health practitioners might agree that rural medical practice has not changed that much over the past century.

Rural Ethical Issues

Certain ethical issues arise more frequently for rural practitioners than for their urban counterparts. In smaller communities, the rural physician is more likely to interact socially with patients outside of the medical context, creating frequent potential for conflict of interest and blurring of roles. A survey with interviews of rural doctors found their biggest ethical concerns to be lack of patient financial resources, patients' failure to understand treatments, insufficient time with patients, and lack of transportation for patients to see a physician (National Rural Bioethics Project 2003).

Researchers have found that small communities experience different health care problems than urban communities. These differences include

- overlapping relationships and conflicting roles among caregivers, patients, and families,
- challenges in preserving patient confidentiality,
- heightened cultural dimensions of health care,
- limited resources and access to health care services and related issues of clinical competence,
- exceptional stresses on caregivers,
- caregivers who must be generalists, and
- limited resources for clinical ethics consultations (Roberts, Battaglia, and Epstein 1999; Roberts et al. 1999).

A lack of relevant resources for the rural practitioner is troublesome. Health professionals working in rural areas found existing ethics materials to be of limited usefulness (National Rural Bioethics Project 2003). Nelson, Lushkov, and Weeks (2006) revealed a limited literature on the topic of ethical issues in rural health care practice. Jecker and Berg reported that rural physicians had different views of the principle of justice than ethicists (most of whom are urban based). They suggest such differences are based in the cultural and resource-restricted realities of rural practice as well as a lack of research about how people use justice in clinical practice (1992, p. 473). Few rural hospitals have ethics committees for deliberation of issues or guided decision making (Cook and Hoas 1999; National Rural Bioethics Project 2003). The differences between rural and urban areas are so complex that some have called for specialized training for physicians working in rural areas (Probst et al. 2002).

REFERENCES

Adams, C. E., Y. Michel, D. DeFrates, and C. F. Corbett. 2001. Effect of locale on health status and direct care time of rural versus urban home health patients. *Journal of Nursing Administration* 31 (5): 244–51.

American Medical Association. 1996. *Socioeconomic characteristics of medical practice 1996.* Chicago: American Medical Association.

Bigbee, J. L. 1991. The concept of hardiness as applied to rural nursing. *Rural Nursing* 1:39–58.

Callahan, D. 1995. Bioethics. In *Encyclopedia of bioethics,* edited by W. T. Reich. New York: Simon & Schuster Macmillan.

Cook, A., and H. Hoas. 1999. Are healthcare ethics committees necessary in rural hospitals? *HEC Forum* 11 (2): 134–39.

Cooper, S. 2000. Consumer/Survivor voice: Rural recovery. Rural mental health. National Association for Rural Mental Health. www.narmh.org/pages/c_srura .html (accessed February 9, 2006).

Cronin, A. J. 1937. *The citadel.* New York: Grosset & Dunlap.

DeJan, E., and W. Yang. 2005. Nevada vital statistics, 2001–2003. Nevada State Health Division. http://health2k.state.nv.us/nihds/publications/VStats/vs0103 .pdf (accessed November 3, 2005).

Diamond, J. 2005. *Collapse.* New York: Penguin.

Eberhardt, M., D. Ingram, D. Makuc, E. R. Pamuk, V. M. Freid, S. B. Harper, C. A. Schoenborn, and H. Xia. 2001. *Urban and rural health chartbook. Health, United States, 2001.* Hyattsville, MD: National Center for Health Statistics.

Frenzen, P. D. 1996. *The Medicare and Medicaid programs in rural America.* U.S. Department of Agriculture.

Frey, W. H. 1995. Elderly demographic profiles of U.S. states: Impacts of "new elderly births," migration, and immigration. *Gerontologist* 35 (6): 761–70.

Gillanders, W. R., and T. F. Buss. 1993. Access to medical care among the elderly in rural northeastern Ohio. *Journal of Family Practice* 37 (4): 349–55.

Hassol, A., G. Gaumer, C. Irvin, J. Grigsby, C. Mintzer, and D. Puskin. 1997. Rural telemedicine data/image transfer methods and purposes of interactive video sessions. *Journal of the American Medical Informatics Association* 4 (1): 36–37.

Jecker, N. S., and A. O. Berg. 1992. Allocating medical resources in rural America: Alternative perceptions of justice. *Social Science and Medicine* 34 (5): 467–74.

Johnson-Webb, K. D., L. D. Baer, and W. M. Gesler. 1997. What is rural? Issues and considerations. *Journal of Rural Health* 13 (3): 253–56.

Kandel, W., and J. Cromartie. 2004. *New patterns of Hispanic settlement in America*. Washington, DC: U.S. Department of Agriculture Economic Research Service.

Klugman, C. M. 2006. Haves and have nots. *American Journal of Bioethics* 6 (2): 63–64.

Long, K. A., and C. Weinert. 1989. Rural nursing: Developing the theory base. *Scholarly Inquiry for Nursing Practice: An International Journal* 3 (2): 113–27.

National Center for Health Statistics. 2004. *Health, United States, 2004, with chartbook on trends in the health of Americans*. Hyattsville, MD: National Center for Health Statistics.

National Rural Bioethics Project. 2003. University of Montana–Missoula. www .umt.edu/bioethics/ (accessed April 2, 2003).

National Rural Health Association. 1998. The role of telemedicine in rural healthcare. www.nrharural.org/advocacy/sub/issuepapers/ipaper7.html (accessed November 28, 2007).

Neimoller, J., B. Ide, and E. Nichols. 2000. Issues in studying health-related hardiness and use of services among older rural adults. *Texas Journal of Rural Health* 8 (1): 35–43.

Nelson, W., G. Lushkov, A. Pomerantz, and W. B. Weeks. 2006. Rural health care ethics: Is there a literature? *American Journal of Bioethics* 6 (2): 44–50.

Office of Management and Budget. 2000. Standards for defining metropolitan and micropolitan statistical areas. *Federal Register* 65 (249):82228–38.

O'Toole, R. 2003. *Census bureau: 94.6 percent of U.S. is rural open space*. Heartland Institute. www.heartland.org/Article.cfm?artId=12402 (accessed November 9, 2005).

Packham, J., and T. Griswold. 2007. *Nevada rural and frontier health data book, 2007 Edition*. Reno: Nevada Office of Rural Health.

Probst, J. C., C. G. Moore, E. G. Baxley, and J. J. Lammie. 2002. Rural-urban differences in visits to primary care physicians. *Family Medicine* 34 (8): 609–15.

Ricketts, T. G., and P. R. Heaphy. 2000. Culture and medicine: Hospitals in rural America. *Western Journal of Medicine* 173 (6): 418–22.

Roberts, L. W., J. Battaglia, and R. S. Epstein. 1999. Frontier ethics: Mental health care needs and ethical dilemmas in rural communities. *Psychiatric Services* 50 (4): 497–503.

Roberts, L. W., J. Battaglia, M. Smithpeter, and R. S. Epstein. 1999. An office on Main Street: Health care dilemmas in small communities. *Hastings Center Report* 29 (4): 28–37.

Rogers, A., and J. Raymer. 2001. Immigration and the regional demographics of the elderly population in the United States. *Journal of Gerontology B: Psychological Sciences and Social Sciences* 56 (1): S44–55.

Singh, G. K., and M. Siahpush. 2002. Increasing rural-urban gradients in U.S. suicide mortality, 1970–1997. *American Journal of Public Health* 92 (7): 1161–67.

Starr, Paul. 1982. *The Social Transformation of American Medicine.* New York: Basic.

United Nations. 2007. Population density and urbanization. http://unstats.un.org (accessed November 12, 2007).

U.S. Census Bureau. 1995. Urban and rural definitions. www.census.gov/population/censusdata/urdef.txt (accessed November 12, 2007).

———. 2002a. Census 2000 urban and rural classification. www.census/gov/geo/wvw/ua/va_2k.htm (accessed April 12, 2007).

———. 2002b. Urban/rural and metropolitan/nonmetropolitan population: 2000, geographic comparison table. http://factfinder.census.gov (accessed November 9, 2005).

———. 2002c. State and County Quick Facts: Alaska. http://quickfacts.census.gov/qfd/states/02000.html (accessed January 29, 2006).

———. 2003. Population in metropolitan and micropolitan statistical areas in alphabetical order and numerical and percent change for the United States and Puerto Rico, 1990 and 2000. www.census.gov/population/cen2000/phc-t29/tab01a.pdf (accessed November 12, 2007).

U.S. Department of Agriculture. 2007. Distance learning, telemedicine money available. *Medical Informatics News,* April 9. www.medinfonews.com/ar/41.htm (accessed November 28, 2007).

U.S. Department of Agriculture, Economic Research Service. 2003. Measuring rurality, What is rural? www.ers.usda.gov/briefing/Rurality/WhatIsRural/ (accessed September 29, 2006).

———. 2004. Measuring rurality: Rural-urban continuum codes. www.ers.usda.gov/briefing/rurality/RuralUrbCon/ (accessed November 12, 2007).

———. 2006. Rural America at a Glance. *Economic Information Bulletin* 18. www.ers.usda.gov/Publications/EIB18 (accessed February 28, 2008).

———. 2007a. Rural population and migration: Trend 2—Nonmetro population growth slows. www.ers.usda.gov/Briefing/Population/Nonmetro.htm (accessed November 12, 2007.)

———. 2007b. *Rural population and migration: Trend 5—Challenges from an aging population.* www.ers.usda.gov/Briefing/Population/Challenges.htm (accessed November 28, 2007).

———. 2007c. Rural population and migration: Trend 5—Diversity increases in nonmetro America. www.ers.usda.gov/Briefing/Population/Diversity.htm (accessed November 12, 2007).

U.S. Department of Health and Human Services. 1996. *Area Resource File.* Washington, DC: Office of Research and Planning, Bureau of Health Professions, Health Resources and Services Administration, Public Health Service, U.S. Department of Health and Human Services.

World Health Organization. 1948. Preamble to the Constitution of the World Health Organization as adopted by the International Health Conference, New York, 19–22 June 1946; signed on 22 July 1946 by the representatives of 61 states. *Official Records of the World Health Organization* 2:100.

Zelarney, P. T., and J. A. Ciarlo. 2000. Defining and Describing Frontier Areas in the United States: An Update. Letter to the Field No. 22. Western Interstate Commission for Higher Education. www.wiche.edu/MentalHealth/Frontier/index .html (accessed January 26, 2006).

PART I

OVERVIEW OF RURALITY AND GENERAL ETHICAL ISSUES

What is unique about rurality and how does it differ from urban-ity? Specific geographic regions have different cultures and values that influence how decisions are made and how health care is delivered. Those providers who practice in rural areas find themselves facing a host of ethical issues, including limited medical ethics resources and a lack of literature on the specific concerns a rural practitioner may face. The rural voice is lacking in the bioethical debate partly because many situations that urban practitioners or bioethicists would view as ethical problems are not defined as "ethical" by rural residents. As a result of such limitations and different definitions, ethical rural resources and time to deal with them are scarce. To the urban ethicist, the question of how to distribute ethical and financial resources to a scattered low-density population creates a challenge of distributive justice and priority setting that has strong policy implications.

CHAPTER 1

Rural-Urban Differences in End-of-Life Care

Reflections on Social Contracts

CHARLES E. GESSERT, M.D., M.P.H.

Interest in regional variation in end-of-life care practices has increased sharply in recent years. The *Dartmouth Atlas of Health Care 1999* concluded that "to the extent that end-of-life issues are addressed in practice, they are resolved in ways that depend on where the patient happens to live, not on the patient's preferences or the power to extend life. The American experience of death varied remarkably from one community to another in 1995–96" (Wennberg and Cooper 1999, p. 176).

Subsequent studies have examined regional variation in the use of specific end-of-life services. Beth A. Virnig and colleagues (2000) documented that the use of hospice services varied widely from community to community and was greater in wealthier areas, urban areas, areas with fewer beds per capita, and areas with higher HMO enrollment. Judith C. Ahronheim and colleagues (2001) demonstrated that tube feeding of cognitively impaired nursing home residents varied markedly from state to state, from 7.4 percent in Maine to 40.2 percent in Mississippi. The *Dartmouth Atlas* also demonstrated that significant regional variation can be seen in many Medicare-reimbursed services in the last six months of life including: likelihood of dying in a hospital, ICU use during terminal hospitalization, average reimbursements for inpatient care, and others (Wennberg and Cooper 1999).

Despite the increased interest in regional variation in end-of-life care, in most studies rural-urban differences are not considered or are examined using a dichotomous metropolitan statistical area (MSA)/non-MSA variable. Few studies provide an analysis of rural-urban differences in their discussion sections. Such differences may be critical, in view of the marked differences between rural and urban cultures.

In previous work, I demonstrated that in Kansas urban nursing home residents with severe cognitive impairment were three times more likely to have a feeding tube near the end of life than their rural counterparts (19.3% versus 6.4%, p<0.001) (Gessert and Calkins 2001). These findings were highly significant for all demographic and clinical subpopulations examined: white and non-white, male and female, those with and without living wills, and those with impairment due to stroke or Alzheimer disease.

At present, the reasons for the marked rural-urban differences in end-of-life care practices are unknown. Certainly access to services plays a part, but many observed differences are too large to be explained by variation in access alone. Rural-urban differences in the relationships between care providers and consumers and rural-urban cultural differences are also thought to be important (Gessert and Calkins 2001). This chapter focuses on the last of these variables—cultural differences—and especially on rural-urban differences in the understanding of social contracts.

Culture and End-of-Life Care Practices

Until a few years ago, the role of culture in end-of-life decision making was "largely ignored within bioethics" (Hern et al. 1998, p. 27). Over the last decade, the interface between culture and the experience of disease and dying has been studied more extensively. In *Medicine and Culture,* Lynn Payer (1996) described the wide range of meanings attached to symptoms, health, and illness in France, West Germany, the United Kingdom, and the United States. Leslie J. Blackhall and colleagues (1995) examined attitudes about discussion of terminal illness among four ethnic groups in Los Angeles County and found marked variation in beliefs about disclosure of terminal diagnosis and whether the patient (as opposed to the family) should make decisions about life-supporting technology. Other studies have documented distinctive patterns of preferences for care near the end of life in ethnic groups such as Asian Americans (Blackhall et al. 1995; Braun 1998; Braun and Nichols 1996; Hern et al. 1998; Long 2000). As one review of cultural issues in death and dying concluded, "Culture is not something apart from us. It is always here, and we, like fish in an ocean, may be blind to the water in which we swim" (Hallenbeck, Goldstein, and Mebane 1996, p. 405).

None of these studies on the role of culture in end-of-life care examined rural-urban cultural differences as a variable. While much has been learned about how traditions rooted in ethnic cultures affect end-of-life care preferences, little has been written on regional or rural-urban cultural differences. In fact, most descriptions of "American" attitudes toward death are in reality descriptions of "urban" attitudes, which may or may not be embraced by rural populations. For example: "At the core of the American value system is the belief that man can master nature, a belief which has motivated the phenomenal technological progress that we now enjoy . . . One result of these beliefs is that most Americans do not really accept death as inevitable; they tend to feel invulnerable" (Howard and Scott 1965, p. 163). This view runs counter to some rural cultural values, as discussed at the end of the chapter.

Mobility and Rural Elderly People: Rurality by Choice

Rural populations are aging due to three demographic factors: the out-migration of the young, the aging-in-place of the resident adults, and the in-migration of elders from larger cities. While this in-migration does not affect all rural areas evenly and has been shown to be a smaller factor than aging in place (Frey 1995; Rogers and Raymer 2001), it nonetheless is an important aspect of contemporary rural culture. The significance lies in the distinctive nature of the migrating elder: "elderly migration is selective of individuals and is undertaken near the age of retirement, the relatively young elderly migrants are, on average, more likely to be married, better educated, wealthier, and healthier than the nonmigrant elderly population that they join" (Rogers and Raymer 2001, p. S51). The reasons given for the migration of elderly people to rural areas include economic advantage, lifestyle advantage, and change in family composition such as the death of a spouse (Hassinger, Hicks, and Godino 1993). The magnitude of the migration of elderly people to rural areas is difficult to determine but is large enough to raise concerns about the burdens on existing service delivery systems (Fuguitt and Beale 1993; Longino and Taplin 1994). The role that access to services plays in elders' decisions to move to rural areas is unknown. We may assume that at least some elders anticipate the tradeoffs inherent in moving to a more rural community. For example, with gains in environment and lifestyle come some losses—less access to some classes of specialized services, such as sophisticated technology and options in health care.

Differences in Health Status

The literature on rural-urban differences in health and use of health care presents a complex picture. Differences in health status are often overshadowed or confounded by differences in age, access to services, attitudes toward health, and personal values. In an analysis of data from the National Longitudinal Mortality Study, researchers found that the lowest risk of mortality was for "persons living in the most rural locales and those living in rural communities in standard metropolitan statistical areas" (Smith et al. 1995, p. 274). The authors concluded that "despite the cumulative urban advantages in terms of social and economic development, urbanization does not necessarily translate into lower mortality risk" (Smith et al. 1995, p. 276). The impression that rural populations have large, unmet health needs derives principally from data on access to services, rather than data on absolute health status: "Contrary to popular belief, there is little evidence that older people living in rural areas of the United States are, as a group, at a health disadvantage when compared with older people living in metropolitan areas" (Thorson and Powell 1992, p. 251).

Rural-urban differences in health status appear to be less significant and less consistent than differences in attitudes toward health and health care (see chaps. 4 and 8). A study of 3,485 elders, after controlling for ill health, found that rural respondents were more likely to report being able to perform activities of daily living. The authors noted that prior research had documented similar differences and had concluded that "nonmetropolitan older adults may possess or project a different set of expectations about aging than do their peers in metropolitan settings and, thus, may be likely to normalize the trajectory of aging in a different way from their metropolitan counterparts" (Rabiner et al. 1997, p. 14).

Another study of health care values among men in the rural Midwest found that respondents did not consistently regard "optimal health" as an independent value and were more inclined to see health in utilitarian terms; that is, "health is being able to work and meet responsibilities"

(Sellers et al. 1999, p. 326). Other studies confirm the centrality of work, independence, and activity in rural values, often overshadowing the value placed on health per se (Larson 1978; White 1977).

A study of rural and urban elders in Nebraska found that although the two groups rated their health equally, the rural elders were much more likely to avoid medical care, leading the authors to conclude that "the real difference . . . was in [how] they construed health and health care. Those in the rural group expressed attitudes of independence and self-reliance, values consistent with concepts of pioneer virtues and responsibility" (Thorson and Powell 1992, p. 259).

Differences in the Use of Health Care

Several investigators have documented significantly lower rates of use of health services in rural areas. An analysis of the National Health Interview Survey's (NHIS) Supplement on Aging found that among 11,101 persons over the age of 65, farm residents used all types of care at lower rates than other subpopulations (Himes and Rutrough 1994). Using data from 6,771 elders in the Medicare Current Beneficiary Survey, after controlling for the availability of health care providers, researchers found that rural beneficiaries used more home health care and fewer physician and hospital services than urban beneficiaries (Dansky et al. 1998). Other investigators have found little difference between use of rural and urban health care by elderly people (Blazer et al. 1995; McConnel and Zetzman 1993). An analysis of data from the National Center for Health Statistics' Longitudinal Study on Aging and the Area Resource File "revealed that the utilization pattern of hospital, nursing home, and physician services was unrelated to either rural or urban residential location or the availability of health resources in the area" (McConnel and Zetzman 1993, p. 270). Similarly, the NHIS study cited above found that the use of hospital stays did not vary with location for most populations (Himes and Rutrough 1994).

For home health care services, rural and urban communities have been found to differ in several ways. An analysis of Medicare databases found that home health use rates were higher in urban areas (Kenney 1993), and several studies have found that fewer rural elders use home health services (Kenney 1993; Nyman et al. 1991). However, Genevieve M. Kenney found that home health care users in rural areas "receive on average three more visits than their urban counterparts" (1993, p. 39).

Rural elders tend to be younger and less disabled at the time of admission to a nursing home (Coward, Netzer, and Mullens 1996; Duncan, Coward, and Gilbert 1997) and have a greater lifetime likelihood of admission than urban elders. However, as in other areas of health care use, the picture here is not simple. Interviews with 1,017 elders regarding preferences for care revealed that while rural elders were more likely to be admitted to nursing homes, they viewed such admission as a less-acceptable option than did their urban counterparts (Peek et al. 1997). Another analysis noted that rural-urban differences in the use of nursing homes hinged on the definitions of *rural* and *urban* that were used (Rabiner, Hipskind, and Randolph 1997).

Differences in Access to Health Care

Comparisons of rural-urban use of health care are confounded by differences in access to services. Several of the studies cited above that found little or no rural-urban difference in the use of services were controlled for access and therefore would not have identified absolute differences in use. A survey of 10,310 households in Minnesota revealed that those in rural areas were more likely to be uninsured or self-insured and that those who were insured had fewer covered benefits and greater likelihood of a deductible than those in urban areas (Hartley, Quam, and Lurie 1994). Despite these differences, rural residents were more likely to have a regular source of care and were less likely to experience delays in obtaining care that they deemed necessary. For Medicare populations, differences in coverage are, of course, much less marked and play a smaller role in access than geographic distance and provider distribution.

A study based on the National Long Term Care Survey examined non-institutional medical, home-, and community-based services used by 4,182 older adults in rural and urban settings (Rabiner 1995). While area of residence was found to be associated with access, the relationship between rural and urban settings was not linear. In fact, access problems were greatest among those in the most rural ("open country") and the most urban (central city) settings and were lowest among those in towns, small cities, and suburbs. This study was designed to identify the factors most strongly associated with having a regular source of care, wanting care but receiving none, and several other measures of access. While rural-urban differences were documented for some aspects of access to care, they were not as powerful as other factors such as family income, age, race, and health status.

Differences in End-of-Life Care

Evidence of rural-urban differences in end-of-life care practices has begun to appear in the medical literature over the last several years. As noted in the introduction to this section, the *Dartmouth Atlas of Health Care 1999* documented marked regional variation in Medicare expenditures for services in the last six months of life but did not focus on rural-urban differences per se (Wennberg and Cooper 1999). More recently, a study done for the Medicare Payment Advisory Commission documented lower average Medicare costs and lower likelihood of using Medicare hospice benefits for rural beneficiaries in the last year of life (Hogan et al. 2000). A follow-up study by the same team found that use of hospice benefits was significantly lower for Medicare decedents in rural areas, even after adjustment for beneficiary characteristics such as age, diagnosis, income, and insurance coverage (Hogan 2001). These findings are consistent with the findings of Virnig and colleagues (2000), summarized above.

Findings from Focus Groups

We convened eight focus groups during 2002 in urban and rural nursing homes in Minnesota to examine end-of-life decision making (Gessert et al. 2006). Each focus group comprised three to nine family members of nursing home residents with advanced dementia. Five rural focus groups were convened in "nonmetro" Minnesota counties that did not have urban centers larger than 20,000 people—according to U.S. Department of Agriculture (USDA) 1993 county codes 6 through 9 (Butler and Beale 1994). The three urban focus groups were held in counties with 1993 USDA county codes 0 through 2 (counties, in major metropolitan areas, with population over 250,000). Nursing home staff members identified potential participants from among families that lived within 50 miles of the nursing home and visited frequently. The rural focus groups comprised predominantly—but not exclusively—lifelong rural residents and were convened in several types of rural community (farming, mining, tourism). We did not distinguish between lifelong residents and in-migrants in the analysis.[1] Following is a summary of some of the principal findings from the focus groups.

Attitudes toward Health Care Providers

The family caregivers who participated in the focus groups provided extensive descriptions of their interactions with and dependency on health care providers, especially nursing homes. However, the nature and style of the interactions between families and health care providers differed in the rural and urban groups. Rural participants demonstrated a more accepting and sympathetic attitude toward the health care providers, often offering explanations about any shortcomings. Their stories reflected their strong belief that they had admitted their relatives to the care of their neighbors and friends. The rural focus groups provided a good deal of anecdotal support for this idea, as we heard frequent references to the multiple points of contact between the rural participants and the staff, visitors, and other residents of their respective nursing homes:

> This has always been a great home, but I've noticed that there's a lot more family involvement, a lot more visitors . . . So, you know, the family is very, very important.

> Very involved . . . They're very good about encouraging that . . . [New speaker]: Yeah, right from the top down.

> You know, most of these people that work here have known me.

> I think it's small enough around here that it's much more personable . . . I mean you really get to know the staff.

Conversely, many urban focus group participants described their own advocacy in strident terms and demonstrated their truculence regarding their elder's "rights" to services and the role the family "had to assume" to ensure that those entitlements were met. Urban families tended to behave as if they were admitting their relatives to the care of strangers, and for most of these families this was the case:

> He would never get fed in a nursing home situation enough to ever exist on.

You learn to play the game . . . You feel like you're fighting the system . . .
You're always on your guard.

Rural participants expected to retain a good deal of hands-on caregiv-
ing responsibility after the admission of their relatives; this was true of
some urban families as well. Urban families tended—more or less uni-
formly—to be more demanding, less sympathetic, and more combative
than their rural counterparts. The research team concluded that these
observed differences were due, at least in part, to the different roles that
nursing homes play in rural and urban communities (see chap. 11). Many
rural nursing homes are major employers and resources in their communities. Perhaps more important, rural families were generally confident that
their elder relatives would receive the kind of care that they would want
to receive because all of the players—residents, staff, and families—shared
a good deal of history and experience. On the other hand, as noted above,
urban families admitted their relatives to more-or-less anonymous institutions and to the care of strangers. Urban families did not generally assume
that "the kind of care that you would want to receive" would be provided
unless they (the admitting relatives) retained a strong advocacy role for
the resident.

Attitudes toward Approaching Death

These families recognized that the endpoint of their relatives' dementia
would be death. Many of the families were comfortable with death and
regarded the prospect of their elders' death with a sense of release and
relief. Conversely, a few of the focus group participants were not ready—
now, or perhaps ever—to express acceptance of death. When asked how
he would know that his mother's "time had come," one participant replied,
"Well, she'll be dead."

A tendency toward greater willingness to accept death was noted among
rural focus group participants. Rural participants described death in neutral or positive terms, often invoking peaceful imagery such as sleep:

Participant 1: Going to sleep and waking up on the other side.

Participant 2: Much better than suffering day after day.

Participant 3: So I'm at peace, and I would like if my dad would lay down
and go sleep and go off to heaven 'cause I know that's where he's gonna go
and everything is all right.

Moderator: So if you could write a script for her?

Participant 4: It would be to just pleasantly decline, and she's lived 96 years and we don't need a lot more.

In the urban focus groups, greater emphasis was placed on delaying or "fighting" death. Many of the participants described their advocacy for medical interventions, even late in the course of dementia:

Participant 5: I felt that . . . the antibiotics he had in the hospital could have maybe been continued longer and that might have sustained him longer.

Participant 6: You have to fight for their rights . . . to live!

The rural-urban differences in attitudes toward death may be due to many factors, including greater rural exposure to the cyclical nature of seasons and crops and more familiarity with the life and death cycles of plants, farm animals, and even extended family. However, this is speculative, as the roots of rural-urban differences in attitudes toward death have not been studied extensively. In these focus groups, however, the differences were appreciable (Gessert, Elliott, and Peden-McAlpine 2006) and even extended to the time frame in which death would be acceptable. Rural participants were often more comfortable in speaking of a proximate death ("tomorrow morning"), whereas many urban participants—while accepting death—tended to be more comfortable with a distant death.

Many of the participants—rural and urban—observed that there are some nursing home residents who do not have anyone to advocate for them. Such residents were the object of concern and pity. Several family caregivers stated that they were inspired in their role as advocates for their relatives by the specter of those who did not have advocates. Additionally, several participants—primarily from rural focus groups—described their activities on behalf of those who did not have friends or family who visited regularly. Urban focus group participants' advocacy on behalf of "those who had no one" tended to be more abstract and less personal; they felt that "someone" ought to help.

A Sense of Community

In 1955, George A. Hillery found that social interaction, common ties, and geographic area were used most often in defining community and that these factors were equally applicable in rural and urban settings. Others who have examined "community" have reached similar conclusions: that community is defined by elements such as "shared emotional connection" (McMillan and Chavis 1986, p. 13), which do not depend primarily on geographic proximity (Glynn 1981). In this light, our observations of rural-urban differences may be seen as reflecting the relative strength of "sense of community" in rural and urban settings.

In the rural focus groups, participants frequently referred to their shared community experiences. They invoked four characteristics of community life: (1) shared life experience over time, such as attending the same schools; (2) interaction in multiple settings, such as work, community, and church; (3) common lifestyles and common values; and (4) interaction among multigenerational extended families. The rural participants also described the multifaceted "connectedness" between the nursing homes and the surrounding communities, consistent with Rowles's description of the "permeability" of a rural nursing home (Rowles, Concotelli, and High 1996). Visitors to the rural nursing homes were likely to know more than one of the residents and might also be familiar with members of the staff or their families. Rural nursing homes were recognized as employers in their communities and as important to the economic life of the area. This network of relationships meant that in rural nursing homes, visitors seemed to find plenty of opportunities to socialize; there was a lot to do and talk about. In summarizing our findings from the eight focus groups, we concluded that rural family members' visits to the nursing home were more *interesting* than their urban counterparts' visits.

In the urban focus groups, participants conveyed their sense that when the elder entered the nursing home, his or her care was placed in the hands of unfamiliar people. The elders would leave much of their history and their community behind when they were admitted. We observed efforts in one of the urban nursing homes to preserve or reestablish the identity of the elders through the posting of short biographies on the doors of the residents' rooms. This practice served to emphasize the uniqueness of each resident. We noted, however, that this approach might be seen as unnecessary in many rural nursing homes, where the life stories of residents are more likely to be recalled without cues.

Clearly, many of the characteristics of the rural communities in our study might be observed in other (nonrural) communities. Further study should be directed at examining the role of "community" in creating stronger—or at least different—types of bonds between the providers and the consumers of health services, especially nursing home services. Such work also has a practical application. If strong community integration could be demonstrated to have a salutary effect on nursing home experiences, steps could be taken to encourage nursing homes to identify and serve well-defined communities, such as those defined by religious or ethnic ties, in rural and urban areas alike.

Reflections on Social Contracts

In recent years, the concept of the social contract has been applied to topics as diverse as marriage, labor relations, taxation, race, party politics, and globalization (Piven and Cloward 1997). In health policy discussions, social contracts have been invoked in the analysis of subjects ranging from the Health Insurance Portability and Accountability Act (HIPAA) (Hiatt 2003), to professionalism (Cruess 2006), to Medicare policy (Geyman 2004, 2006). Despite the wide—and occasionally fanciful—application of the concept of social contracts in diverse arguments, the concept remains useful. At root, discussions of social contracts are discussions of the tacit understandings that bind communities together. In this sense, social contracts may be useful in examining the differences between rural and urban cultures, and rural and urban end-of-life care.

Rural and Urban Cultures: Historical Considerations

Today, rural U.S. communities are diverse, with economies based on industries ranging from agriculture and forestry to tourism and retirement. However, the agrarian roots of rural culture are strong. In his writings on the family farm in America, Victor Davis Hanson (1996) emphasizes the historical role of the agrarian voice: "Whatever one thinks now of Western culture, he should at least recognize that its foundations—economic, social, political and military—originated in the countryside . . . [The agrarian] has been for twenty-five hundred years the critical counter voice to a material and uniform culture . . . Is there another . . . whose voice says no to popular tastes, no to the culture of the suburb, no to the urban enclave, no to the gated estate?" (pp. x–xii).

At the time of the American Revolution, 95 percent of the U.S. population was rural, and Thomas Jefferson considered the "cultivators of the earth" to be "the most valuable citizens" of the new republic (Carlson 2000, p. 1). Most writers on rural culture—from Jefferson to contemporary sociologists—have emphasized independence and self-sufficiency as the core values that characterize rural culture. The full picture of rural culture is more complex and less romantic. In addition to valuing independence and self-sufficiency, or perhaps as an extension of these values, agrarians are likely to be skeptical, stubborn, resistant to change, and unreceptive to ideas that come from outside of their common experience (Hanson 1996). Hanson points to the divergence of contemporary rural and urban cultures and to the determination of the farmer to preserve a distinctive way of life: "In the farmers' mind, given their pessimistic views of urban America in the late twentieth century, there is no other avenue to ensure their children a moral future, save by putting them on the land and putting them to work. Only that way, for the rest of their lives will they have a house, not houses, have a job, not jobs, have a town, not towns, have a family, not families, know where they are born and where they will die" (1996, p. xiii).

While one cannot attribute this "agrarian voice" to all who live in rural areas, especially in view of demographic changes in rural America, it would also be a mistake to dismiss rural values and culture as anachronisms. Rural life has been and remains a distinctive experience, one that is increasingly experienced by choice rather than as an accident of birthplace (Carlson 2000; Coward and Rathbone-McCuan 1985; Hynson 1975; Lee and Cassidy 1985; Lee and Lassey 1980).

Social Contracts and Health Care

Our observations of rural caregivers are consistent with the findings described by Katherine Brown (1994) in "Outside the Garden of Eden: Rural Values and Healthcare Reform." She observed that rural and urban people are likely to be similar in their conviction that elderly and indigent people should be cared for, but they may envision and invoke different "social contracts" as rationales for the care. Rural people tend to think of the provision of care to those who cannot care for themselves as charity (i.e., a gift that is voluntarily given as part of the social contract or social fabric of the community). One becomes "eligible" to receive this charity by virtue of one's role (e.g., a lifelong teacher in a local school) or status (e.g., an elder who worked hard all her life). Because all services are gifts, under this model, the *need* of the recipient is an important part of the equation because a gift to someone who does not need it is indeed empty. The provision of care, even if done under contract and with a weekly paycheck, never wholly loses the sense that it is an act of charity. Urban people, on the other hand, tend to recognize the concept of "entitlement," which is wholly foreign to the rural mind-set. In the urban way of thinking, by virtue of paying taxes (or by virtue of citizenship itself) one is *entitled* to a range of services, regardless of need. The entitlement is there and may have to be defended and demanded, but it is "owned" by the recipient. Providers of care to urban recipients are providing a service that the recipient is entitled to; there is no gift in the equation.

Brown (1994) found that rural respondents did not view health care as a "right" or "entitlement" but as a service that is provided on the basis of compassion and rooted in the reciprocal relationships (neighborliness) within the community. This distinction is particularly relevant to end-of-life care services, in that it places emphasis on the need for (or utility of) the service in question. Whereas the need for and utility of a service are not essential factors in a transaction based on entitlement, they are core considerations in the provision of a service that is viewed as a gift and is based on compassion (the rural view). For these rural respondents, the merits of the service recipient and the manifest need for the service were important determinants in health care decision making.

The implications of these rural-urban cultural differences for end-of-life decision making may be significant. To the degree that health care services are seen as gifts, rather than entitlements, the decision to provide the service must meet several tests not imposed by the more principle-based abstract reasoning that guides much of our dominant (essentially urban) medical culture. Most importantly, the donor (or family decision maker) retains a large role in assessing the potential benefit of the service because that is the basis for its value as a gift.

Although rural U.S. populations are no longer predominantly agrarian, an agrarian mentality continues to be an important part of rural culture and may mediate some aspects of the effect of rural culture on end-of-life care preferences. Agrarian workers—those who work the land—have occupied a distinctive niche in society for thousands of years (Hanson 1999). As noted above, the "agrarian idea" that such rural populations defend within a culture may be characterized as conservative, practical, skeptical about innovation, and resistant to change (Hanson 1996). An agrarian voice in a culture serves as a "brake" on the introduction of new ideas, especially ideas that run counter to common experience, conventional wisdom, and common sense (Buttel and Flinn 1975; Flinn and Johnson 1974; Larson 1978).

Few studies in the health or sociology literature distinguish between agrarian and nonagrarian rural communities. This distinction may be important, especially in contemporary America, for clearly all that is rural is not necessarily agrarian. If differences between rural and urban end-of-life care practices can be documented, it will be important to consider agrarian and nonagrarian rural areas separately in further research on location and end-of-life care.

Implications for Ethical Practices

As a nation, we are struggling to achieve a better balance in our end-of-life care services: a better balance between curative care and palliative care, between preserving life and accepting death, between quantity of life and quality of life. Our rural areas may represent a repository of traditions, of ways of thinking, which have served us well in the past and continue to be used today. These rural traditions may be instructive to the nation as a whole. They may provide insights into the values and relationships that serve to limit the use of aggressive medical interventions near the end of life. To take full advantage of this resource, our predominantly urban culture will need to put aside some of its assumptions and some of its condescension regarding rural culture. Future research should be directed at teasing out distinctive rural end-of-life care practices and principles and, it is to be hoped, illuminating how end-of-life care for all can be improved.

NOTE

1. This research was supported by the National Institute on Aging (Grant #1 R03 AG21214-01) and the Duluth Clinic Education and Research Foundation.

REFERENCES

Ahronheim, J. C., M. Mulvihill, C. Sieger, P. Park, and B. E. Fries. 2001. State practice variations in the use of tube feeding for nursing home residents with severe cognitive impairment. *Journal of the American Geriatric Society* 49 (2): 148–52.

Blackhall, L. J., S. T. Murphy, G. Frank, V. Michel, and S. Azen. 1995. Ethnicity and attitudes toward patient autonomy. *Journal of the American Medical Association* 274 (10): 820–25.

Blazer, D. G., L. R. Landerman, G. Fillenbaum, and R. Horner. 1995. Health services access and use among older adults in North Carolina: Urban vs. rural residents. *American Journal of Public Health* 85 (10):1384–90.

Braun, K. L. 1998. Do Hawaii residents support physician-assisted death? A comparison of five ethnic groups. *Hawaii Medical Journal* 57 (6): 529–34.

Braun, K. L., and R. Nichols. 1996. Cultural issues in death and dying. *Hawaii Medical Journal* 55 (12): 260–64.

Brown, K. H. 1994. Outside the Garden of Eden: Rural values and healthcare reform. *Cambridge Quarterly of Healthcare Ethics* 3 (3): 329–37.

Butler, M. A., and C. L. Beale. 1994. *Rural-urban continuum codes for metro and nonmetro counties, 1993.* Washington, DC: U.S. Department of Agriculture.

Buttel, F. H., and W. L. Flinn. 1975. Sources and consequences of agrarian values in American society. *Rural Sociology* 40 (2): 134–51.

Carlson, A., ed. 2000. *The new Agrarian mind: The movement toward decentralist thought in twentieth-century America.* New Brunswick, NJ: Transaction Publishers.

Coward, R. T., J. K. Netzer, and R. A. Mullens. 1996. Residential differences in the incidence of nursing home admissions across a six-year period. *Journal of Gerontology B: Psychological Sciences and Social Sciences* 51 (5): S258–67.

Coward, R. T., and E. Rathbone-McCuan. 1985. Delivering health and human services to the elderly in rural society. In *The elderly in rural society*, edited by R. T. Coward and G. R. Lee. New York: Springer.

Cruess, S. R. 2006. Professionalism and medicine's social contract with society. *Clinical Orthopaedics and Related Research* 449:170–76.

Dansky, K. H., D. Brannon, D. G. Shea, J. Vasey, and R. Dirani. 1998. Profiles of hospital, physician, and home health service use by older persons in rural areas. *Gerontologist* 38 (3): 320–30.

Duncan, R. P., R. T. Coward, and G. H. Gilbert. 1997. Rural-urban comparisons of age and health at the time of nursing home admission. *Journal of Rural Health* 13 (2): 118–25.

Flinn, W. L., and D. E. Johnson. 1974. Agrarianism among Wisconsin farmers. *Rural Sociology* 39 (2): 187–204.

Frey, W. H. 1995. Elderly demographic profiles of U.S. states: Impacts of "new elderly births," migration, and immigration. *Gerontologist* 35 (6): 761–70.

Fuguitt, G. V., and C. L. Beale. 1993. The changing concentration of the older non-metropolitan population, 1960–90. *Journal of Gerontology* 48 (6): S278–88.

Gessert, C. E., and D. R. Calkins. 2001. Rural-urban differences in end-of-life care: The use of feeding tubes. *Journal of Rural Health* 17 (1): 16–24.

Gessert, C. E., B. A. Elliott, and C. Peden-McAlpine. 2006. Family decision making for nursing home residents with dementia: Rural-urban differences. *Journal of Rural Health* 22 (1):1–8.

Gessert, C. E., I. V. Haller, R. L. Kane, and H. Degenholtz. 2006. Rural-urban differences in medical care for nursing home residents with severe dementia at the end of life. *Journal of the American Geriatrics Society* 54 (8): 1199–205.

Geyman, J. 2006. *Shredding the social contract: The privatization of Medicare.* Monroe, ME: Common Courage Press.

Geyman, J. P. 2004. Privatization of Medicare: Toward disentitlement and betrayal of a social contract. *International Journal of Health Services* 34 (4): 573–94.

Glynn, T. J. 1981. Psychological sense of community: Measurement and application. *Human Relations* 34:789–818.

Hallenbeck, J., M. K. Goldstein, and E. W. Mebane. 1996. Cultural considerations of death and dying in the United States. *Clinics in Geriatric Medicine* 12 (2): 393–406.

Hanson, V. D. 1996. *Fields without dreams: Defending the Agrarian idea.* New York: Free Press.

———. 1999. *The other Greeks: The family farm and the Agrarian roots of Western civilization.* Berkeley and Los Angeles: University of California Press.

Hartley, D., L. Quam, and N. Lurie. 1994. Urban and rural differences in health insurance and access to care. *Journal of Rural Health* 10 (2): 98–108.

Hassinger, E. W., L. L. Hicks, and V. Godino. 1993. A literature review of health issues of the rural elderly. *Journal of Rural Health* 9 (1): 68–75.

Hern, H. E., Jr., B. A. Koenig, L. J. Moore, and P. A. Marshall. 1998. The difference that culture can make in end-of-life decision making. *Cambridge Quarterly of Healthcare Ethics* 7 (1): 27–40.

Hiatt, R. A. 2003. HIPAA: The end of epidemiology, or a new social contract? *Epidemiology* 14 (6): 637–39.

Hillery, G. A. 1955. Definitions of community: Areas of agreement. *Rural Sociology* 20:111–23.

Himes, C. L., and T. S. Rutrough. 1994. Differences in the use of health services by metropolitan and nonmetropolitan elderly. *Journal of Rural Health* 10 (2): 80–88.

Hogan, C. 2001. *Medicare beneficiaries' access to hospice services in rural areas: An initial analysis.* Washington, DC: Medical Payment Advisory Commission.

Hogan, C., J. Lynn, J. Gabel, J. Lunney, A. O'Mara, and A. Wilkinson. 2000. *Medicare beneficiaries' costs and use of care in the last year of life.* Washington, DC: Medical Payment Advisory Commission.

Howard, A., and R. A. Scott. 1965. Cultural values and attitudes toward death. *Journal of Existentialism* 6 (22): 161–74.

Hynson, L. M. 1975. Rural-urban differences in satisfaction among the elderly. *Rural Sociology* 40 (1): 64–66.

Kenney, G. M. 1993. Rural and urban differentials in Medicare home health use. *Health Care Finance Review* 14 (4): 39–57.

Larson, O. F. 1978. Values and beliefs of rural people. In *Rural U.S.A.: Persistence and change,* edited by T. R. Ford. Ames: Iowa State University Press.

Lee, G. R., and M. L. Cassidy. 1985. Family and kin relations of the rural elderly. In *The elderly in rural society,* edited by R. T. Coward and G. R. Lee. New York: Springer.

Lee, G. R., and M. L. Lassey. 1980. Rural-urban differences among the elderly: Economic, social, and subjective factors. *Journal of Social Issues* 36 (2): 62–74.

Long, S. O. 2000. Living poorly or dying well: Cultural decisions about life-supporting treatment for American and Japanese patients. *Journal of Clinical Ethics* 11 (3): 236–50.

Longino, C. F., Jr., and I. M. Taplin. 1994. How does the mobility of the elderly affect health care delivery in the U.S.A.? *Aging (Milano)* 6 (6): 399–409.

McConnel, C. E., and M. R. Zetzman. 1993. Urban/rural differences in health service utilization by elderly persons in the United States. *Journal of Rural Health* 9 (4): 270–80.

McMillan, D. W., and D. M. Chavis. 1986. Sense of community: A definition and theory. *Journal of Community Psychology* 14:6–23.

Nyman, J. A., A. Sen, B. Y. Chan, and P. P. Commins. 1991. Urban/rural differences in home health patients and services. *Gerontologist* 31 (4): 457–66.

Payer, L. 1996. *Medicine and culture.* New York: Henry Holt & Co.

Peek, C. W., R. T. Coward, G. R. Lee, and B. A. Zsembik. 1997. The influence of community context on the preferences of older adults for entering a nursing home. *Gerontologist* 37 (4): 533–42.

Piven, F. F., and R. A. Cloward. 1997. *The breaking of the American social compact.* New York: New Press.

Rabiner, D. J. 1995. Patterns and predictors of noninstitutional health care utilization by older adults in rural and urban America. *Journal of Rural Health* 11 (4): 259–73.

Rabiner, D. J., M. G. Hipskind, and R. K. Randolph. 1997. Are rural elders healthier and happier upon admission to a nursing home setting? *Journal of Clinical Geropsychology* 3 (4): 299–319.

Rabiner, D. J., T. R. Konrad, G. H. DeFriese, J. Kincade, S. L. Bernard, A. Woomert, T. Arcury, and M. G. Ory. 1997. Metropolitan versus nonmetropolitan differences in functional status and self-care practice: Findings from a national sample of community-dwelling older adults. *Journal of Rural Health* 13 (1): 14–28.

Rogers, A., and J. Raymer. 2001. Immigration and the regional demographics of the elderly population in the United States. *Journal of Gerontology B: Psychological Sciences and Social Sciences* 56 (1): S44–55.

Rowles, G. D., J. A. Concotelli, and D. M. High. 1996. Community integration of a rural nursing home. *Journal of Applied Gerontology* 15 (2): 188–201.

Sellers, S. C., M. D. Poduska, L. H. Propp, and S. I. White. 1999. The health care meanings, values, and practices of Anglo-American males in the rural Midwest. *Journal of Transcendental Nursing* 10 (4): 320–30.

Smith, M. H., R. T. Anderson, D. D. Bradham, and C. F. Longino, Jr. 1995. Rural and urban differences in mortality among Americans 55 years and older: Analysis of the National Longitudinal Mortality Study. *Journal of Rural Health* 11 (4): 274–85.

Thorson, J. A., and F. C. Powell. 1992. Rural and urban elderly construe health differently. *Journal of Psychology* 126 (3): 251–60.

Virnig, B. A., S. Kind, M. McBean, and E. Fisher. 2000. Geographic variation in hospice use prior to death. *Journal of the American Geriatrics Society* 48 (9): 1117–25.

Wennberg, J. E., and M. M. Cooper, eds. 1999. *The quality of medical care in the United States: A report on the Medicare program—The Dartmouth atlas of health care 1999.* Chicago: AHA Press.

White, M. A. 1977. Values of elderly differ in rural setting. *Generations* 1 (4): 6–7.

CHAPTER 2

The Challenges of Rural Health Care

WILLIAM A. NELSON, PH.D.

In the romantic comedy *Doc Hollywood,* Michael J. Fox portrays a young, aspiring plastic surgeon from Washington, D.C. While driving his Porsche cross-country to Beverly Hills, where a lucrative practice awaits, Fox's character manages to wreck his car, destroying some property in a small, isolated rural community and, as it soon appears, his entire Southern California dream as well. A local judge sentences him to 30 days of providing medical coverage to the local community while the town's lone physician takes a much-needed vacation. What ensues is a predictably funny, romantic transformation for the young doctor as well as the local residents.

The film captures in a light-hearted yet all too realistic manner the influence of the rural context on the delivery of health care. Fox's character gradually and painfully experiences the limitations and rewards that inevitably accompany his journey into becoming that stereotypic "country doc" with whom we are all familiar. Instead of feeling discouraged by the protagonist's constant challenges and the limitations presented by his professional isolation, stressful workload as a one-person clinic, and unexpected situations, viewers are uplifted by the depth of his growing relationships and inspired by the level of his commitment to the residents living in this remote, previously foreign, community. Though created in the tradition of happy endings, *Doc Hollywood* offers viewers a comedic glimpse into a world presumed to be largely unknown and rarely understood by those who live in metropolitan and urban settings (see part 2).

The discipline of health care ethics or bioethics, as some may argue, has evolved historically from many wide-ranging areas of focus. The *Encyclopedia of Bioethics* has noted four overlapping areas of inquiry: theoretical, clinical, regulatory and policy, and cultural (Callahan 1995). Theoretical health care ethics deals with the foundations of moral reasoning that are applied to a variety of health care topics. Clinical ethics refers to challenges in individual patient care. Regulatory and policy health care ethics is the organizational and legal reflection of health care–related ethical questions. Cultural health care ethics refers to an effort to systematically relate health care ethics to the cultural and social context in which ethical conflicts arise. One of the subgroups of inquiry for cultural health care ethics is the rural setting.

Rural health care ethics is generally characterized by two fundamental features. First, it focuses on how rural settings can affect and shape ethical conflicts and their responses. Few researchers or practitioners recognize how rural settings may affect the application of ethical guidelines to ethical conflicts (Kitchens et al. 1998). Second, health care ethics has been stirred by new technology and research—such as stem cell research, human reproductive technology, or genetics—which tend to be developed in nonrural academic medical centers (Hardwig 2006), whereas most of the rural health care ethics issues tend to focus on the less glamorous issues of providing basic care within the provider-patient encounter (Klugman 2006).

After briefly discussing the imprecise definition of *rural,* this chapter describes some of the unique and distinguishing characteristics of the rural setting and how they differ from metropolitan and urban settings. A discussion of how rural settings can influence ethical challenges for health care professionals is followed by a review of some of the limitations of ethics resources for rural health care providers. Finally, this chapter offers some practical recommendations for future directions and focus of rural health care ethics.

What Is Meant by *Rural*?

To fully appreciate the magnitude of rural health care ethics, we need to operationally define our target population—rural communities. Currently, there exists no standardized and uniform definition of *rural.* For example, between 1993 and 1995, contributors to the *Journal of Rural Health* used no fewer than 26 different definitions (Johnson-Webb, Baer, and Gesler 1997). Definitions used to classify rural populations can vary dramatically, from simple—such as those calculating people living within a specified geographic area—to complex—for example, definitions taking into account social relationships and community lifestyles. These variations in definition can produce different estimates of the U.S. rural population and might lead to significant implications for practicing clinicians, ethicists, policy planners, lawmakers, health care researchers, and, most importantly, rural residents (Bushy 1993, 1994; Johnson-Webb, Baer, and Gesler 1997; U.S. Census Bureau 1995, 2002).

In the mid-1990s, a comprehensive categorization scheme, the Rural-Urban Community Area (RUCA) classification system, was developed and continues to be increasingly used in health care research (WWAMI Rural Health Research Center 2006). For the purposes of this chapter, we define rural communities as those living in "small towns and isolated rural areas" according to the rural-urban continuum specified by the four-tiered RUCA classification (Washington State Department of Health 2007). Consequently, based on population data collected at the zip code level from the 2000 U.S. Census, approximately 13 percent of the U.S. population lived in rural communities (Nelson and Weeks 2006). Some authors have used larger numbers to denote the extent of rural communities: "approximately 62 million people, roughly 20–23% of the United States' population, live in rural communities distributed over three-quarters of our country's mass" (Nelson et al. 2007, p. 136; Ricketts 2000; Roberts, Battaglia, and Epstein 1999; Institute of Medicine 2005). The rural population numbers based on the 2000 census differ because of the classification scheme used. Despite those differences the point remains constant—rural communities encompass a significant portion of the U.S. population. Throughout this chapter, I discuss and cite references that have used different methodologies and classifications to define rural populations.

Rural Characteristics

In addition to a small population density and long geographical distance to a large population center, there are many general characteristics common to rural communities. The differences between rural and urban areas—in economic status, social, health-related, and cultural factors, as well as the role of medical professionals—which have implications for health care and health care ethics have been and continue to be studied (see chap. 1). Some of these differences are highlighted and discussed here in a manner similar to my earlier papers (Nelson et al. 2007; Nelson and Schmidek 2008).

Limited Economic Resources

On average, the rural population has a lower income per capita and higher rate of poverty compared to the urban population (Nelson and Pomerantz 1992a; Ricketts 2000; Roberts, Battaglia, and Epstein 1999; Roberts et al. 1999; see also chap. 10). Rural residents are also more likely to be underinsured or uninsured, further increasing the financial hardship of interacting with the health care system (Bushy 1994).

Health Indicators

Compared to urban residents, rural residents tend to have poorer overall health. They are more likely to have a chronic or life-threatening disease (Roberts, Battaglia, and Epstein 1999; Roberts et al. 1999) and to face significant mental health issues, including substance abuse and seasonal affective disorder (Bushy 1994). Rural populations also have higher rates of infant mortality (National Center for Health Statistics 2001b) and suicide (National Center for Health Statistics 2001c) and encounter a higher prevalence of environmental and occupational hazards (Gamm et al. 2003; Roberts, Battaglia, and Epstein 1999; Roberts et al. 1999).

Rural communities have a higher proportion of residents, especially adolescents and elderly people, who require more health services (National Center for Health Statistics 2001a; Purtilo 1987; Ricketts 2000). A large study of U.S. veterans found those living in rural settings had worse overall health-related quality of life scores than their urban counterparts (Weeks et al. 2004).

Limited Availability of Health Services

In contrast to residents of urban areas, rural residents tend to be served by fewer health care providers, enjoy a more limited scope of medical services, and experience greater distances when accessing different points of the health care delivery system (see chaps. 4 and 6). With the exception of family practitioners, shortages of a variety of health care professionals have also been documented and include nurses, social workers, dentists, home-based providers, and mental health professionals. Mental health services are especially limited for people living in rural communities (Gamm et al. 2003; Ricketts 2000; Roberts, Battaglia, and Epstein 1999; Roberts et al. 1999). While there are underserved communities throughout the country, the majority of shortages of health professionals are in rural counties.

Health care facilities in rural areas generally are small and frequently provide a limited scope of services. Critical Access Hospitals (CAH) frequently provide health care services to residents of rural communities. To foster the economic solvency and availability of hospitals in rural settings, Congress created in 1997 a CAH designation that allows states to license small hospitals with a maximum of 25 acute beds to be reimbursed on a cost-basis method. As of October 5, 2006, there were 1,284 CAHs, many serving rural populations (Flex Monitoring Team 2006). Geographic isolation and limited services can also force rural health care providers to make decisions based on clinical impression more than the most up-to-date specialty knowledge or diagnostic technology (Cook, Hoas, and Guttmannova 2002; Nelson and Pomerantz 1992b; Roberts, Battaglia, and Epstein 1999; Roberts et al. 1999; Rourke and Rourke 1998).

Given the lack of public transportation, challenging roads, and environmental and climatic barriers, such as oceans, mountain ranges, or extreme weather conditions (Cook and Hoas 2000), rural residents may be adversely limited, and even prohibited, from accessing health care services due to geographic distance (Butler and Beale 1994; Nelson and Pomerantz 1992a; Nelson and Schmidek 2008). These obstacles often make transfer to urban care centers difficult or impossible. In addition, patients may be reluctant to seek care at a faraway facility when they know that family and friends are less likely to be able to provide support because of the distance. In comparisons to urban populations, the conclusion that rural populations are both underserved and vulnerable seems justified.

Sociocultural factors also play an important role in shaping rural health and health care, including the relative homogeneity of individual rural communities, reliance on informal support networks, and overlapping social roles and relationships.

Shared Culture and Values

Health care in the rural United States is deeply affected by the cultural values and beliefs of rural communities. While there is no such thing as a common "rural culture," such communities do tend to be culturally distinct from urban centers. There is usually less diversity within rural communities—although there is considerable diversity *across* rural communities from one part of the country to another—and rural residents tend to share more values than their urban counterparts (Nelson 2004; Roberts, Battaglia, and Epstein 1999; Roberts et al. 1999; see chap. 1). As a result of geographic factors like distance from population centers and the relative cultural homogeneity of rural communities, "living in small towns or sparsely populated areas as opposed to living in more populated areas creates some unique experiences for those residents, especially in regard to health care" (Bushy 1994, p. 255).

The personal and shared cultural values of rural residents affect how they perceive illness, when and from whom they seek health care, their attitudes toward and acceptance of caregivers, how they think about informed consent, and what kinds of treatment decisions they make. Particularly common in rural settings are several general values that influence health care decision making. These values include self-reliance and self-care, use of informal supports (i.e., neighbors, family, and church), a strong work ethic, and defining health and illness not so much in medical terms as in reference to whether one can or cannot work. The greater the extent to which values are shared within the community, the more strongly those values are likely to influence health care relationships and practices. And the more that pervasive community values and perceptions differ from the professional perspective and ethos of clinicians, the more likely it is that ethical conflicts will arise.

Informal Support Networks

Low population density, isolation, limited health care resources and services, and the close-knit nature of rural communities affect the availability and use of public support for health-related needs (see chap. 7). When "compared to urban residents, rural residents historically have preferred and relied on informal social support systems, thereby enhancing their self-reliance" (Bushy 1994, p. 257). Rural residents tend to turn first to families and friends when support is needed. These informal, nonfinancial relationships are usually reciprocal, implicitly based on the understanding that the recipient of services now will later be repaid in kind. Support services provided by community organizations, such as the Grange, churches, or civic organizations, buttress the efforts of family and friends. A third level of support consists of more formal services sponsored by government agencies.

Overlapping Professional-Patient Relationships

Due to the geographical and social structure of rural communities, rural health care providers commonly participate in multiple relationships with members of the community (Bushy 1994; Nelson and Pomerantz 1992a; Roberts, Battaglia, and Epstein 1999; Roberts et al. 1999; chaps. 5 and 7). Practicing medicine in a small setting generally means living and working in the same place (i.e., being "part of the community"). A dominant theme for rural health care professionals is one of familiarity. Everyone knows one another, and certainly everyone knows the community's physician and/or nurse. There is no escaping the role of physician or nurse. Because rural health care professionals are more likely to interact outside their professional realm with members of the community in which they practice—for example, as members of the same church or a community organization—these multiple relationships can enhance and complicate patient care.

This ongoing contact gives health professionals a rare opportunity to know their patients in depth as well as to understand their values and perspectives. The provider-patient relationship is formed in the examining room and in the general store. Such a process allows rural providers a knowledge of their patients that is unlikely in most other settings; these are "relationships that, though they may challenge sterile guidelines made by medical associations, are nonetheless fruitful" (Kullnat 2007, p. 344).

Caregiver Stress

One additional characteristic of the rural setting that can pose distinctive challenges for health care professionals is caregiver stress. The combination of professional isolation, overlapping relationships, immense clinical responsibilities, and emotional and physical exhaustion commonly lead to significant stress. Rural providers also tend to have limited resources to help cope with such stress (Roberts, Battaglia, and Epstein 1999; Roberts et al. 1999). Coupled with the rural value of self-reliance, providers either just stoically accept the stress or burn out.

Ethical Conflicts in Rural Health Care

Like their urban counterparts, health care professionals in rural settings face a variety of ethical questions. But while the fundamental ethical conflicts or questions may be similar across settings, rural settings influence those questions in unique ways (Nelson and Schmidek 2008). The following cases illustrate ethical questions common to rural physicians, including boundaries in the professional-patient relationship, privacy and confidentiality, conflicts of interest, ability to pay, competing professional obligations, disease stigma, and providing care beyond one's area of training when needed services are not otherwise available.

Case 1. A rural psychiatrist, also the chair of the local church's executive council, discovers during a therapy session that one of his patients, the church's youth director, has a significant addiction problem.

Case 2. A primary care provider working in a small, remote, critical access hospital suspects that a patient has ovarian cancer. The provider refers the patient to a distant, large medical center for further assessment and treatment. After several overnight trips to the distant medical center, the patient returns to the primary care provider and indicates that she has been diagnosed with ovarian cancer but is not willing to travel to the medical center for treatment. The patient insists that she wants to receive care at the small hospital, despite the lack of specialized services (see chap. 11).

Case 3. A family physician has provided care to a patient for smoking-related chronic obstructive pulmonary disease for several years. However, the patient has missed her last two appointments. When the physician speaks with the patient after church, the patient indicates that her spouse lost his job as a logger and no longer has health insurance. Refusing to accept any form of government assistance, the patient offers to clean the physician's home and office in exchange for health care services (Nelson and Schmidek 2008).

Case 4. A family physician cares for a neighbor for a minor farming-related injury. The patient is depressed and tearful but refuses to discuss it. The physician encourages the patient to see a mental health professional for further assessment and, if needed, to receive treatment for depression. The patient acknowledges feeling depressed but does not want help, stating, "If people see my truck at the shrink's office everyone will know I have that type of problem—that I'm crazy" (Nelson and Schmidek 2008). The patient also tells his physician not to make any reference to depression in the medical record because his cousin works in the doctor's office (Nelson and Schmidek 2008).

Case 5. A patient in the second trimester of pregnancy is receiving prenatal care from her primary care physician—a single mother practicing in a small, isolated village for whom the patient provides child care. The patient is showing early signs of mild gestational hypertension that could justify a recommendation for regular bed rest. The physician worries that her recommendation would go unheeded because of the community's work ethic, but she's also concerned that if the recommendation is heeded, she will likely lose child care for her three-year old, which will have a devastating effect on her ability to practice medicine.

As illustrated in these cases, familiarity and overlapping relationships dominate life in rural communities. Physicians are also close neighbors and members of the school board; patients are bankers and tradespeople. Health care facilities are often among the largest employers in some small towns, so it is not uncommon for a patient's relative or neighbor to be a member of the health care professional's staff or even the billing clerk who records diagnoses. In small, close-knit communities, where everyone knows everyone else, there is often little privacy (Cook and Hoas 2001; Kullnat 2007; Nelson 2004; Nelson and Pomerantz 1992b; Purtilo 1987; Purtilo and Sorrell 1986; Roberts et al. 1999; Roberts and Dyer 2004), which can lead to ethical conflicts (Campbell and Gordon 2003; Glover 2001; Henderson 2000; Jennings 1992; Schank 1998; Spiegel 1990).

In rural settings, ethical conflicts involving boundary issues are inevitable, such as in Case 1 (Cook and Hoas 2000, 2001; Kullnat 2007; Larson 2001; Miller 1994; Nelson 2004; Nelson and Schmidek 2008; Purtilo 1987; Purtilo and Sorrell 1986; Roberts, Battaglia, and Epstein 1999; Roberts et al. 1999; Roberts and Dyer 2004, see chaps. 7 and 8). If the provider disengages from dual relations, the patient might feel a sense of rejection or an erosion of trust, thus resulting in a less productive clinical atmosphere (Purtilo and Sorrell 1986). Competing obligations as physician and church council member force the clinician to weigh whether to take administrative action against the youth director based on privileged medical knowledge. Any decision will have ramifications for the clinician's patients, the church, and others in the community. Ethical conflicts involving caring for individual patients while trying to balance competing needs of other patients and the community are routine for rural clinicians. With no other caregivers available, patients, too, are often unable to avoid such potential conflicts.

Case 2 highlights common ethical issues faced by rural physicians whose patients may resist or refuse transfer to urban, tertiary care centers, often because they mistrust or fear this unfamiliar setting (Nelson and Pomerantz 1992b). When confronted with a mentally competent patient who refuses care that the clinician believes is essential, the clinician must decide how aggressively to try to persuade the patient to seek treatment at the distant urban medical center. If the patient continues to refuse the referral, the clinician must address the burden of providing the needed care. Both physicians and nurses in rural communities have expressed concerns that they compromise quality because they must practice outside their area of training (Cook and Hoas 2000, 2001; Cook, Hoas, and Joyner 2000; Larson 2001; Turner, Marquis, and Burman 1996; see chaps. 5 and 8) as well as compromise professional ethical norms. The ethical issue is accentuated by legal concerns when professionals believe they are practicing outside their scope of competence.

Case 3 highlights the influence of common rural culture on ethics conflicts. Rural patients tend to avoid government support and rely on their families or churches as the primary support system (Bushy 1994). The acceptance of bartering in rural culture can challenge professional ethical standards, and the clinician's failure to recognize or respect local values can lead to an ethical conflict. Additional issues arise when the clinician overemphasizes community values at the cost of compromising professional or personal values (Roberts et al. 1999; Roberts and Dyer 2004). Unfortunately, the medical professional's ethical guidelines seldom provide adequate insight into the role of rural cultural beliefs in sound ethical decision making.

The case also reflects how rural health care professionals regularly encounter situations where they must decide whether to provide needed care with little or no reimbursement, potentially jeopardizing both the patients' health and the provider's overall practice (Cook, Hoas, and Guttmannova 2002; Ricketts 2000; Turner, Marquis, and Burman 1996) and their standing within the community. Not providing needed services is a difficult decision because it may be contrary to community values and the perceived role of the clinician. Because everyone in the community knows the physician, such decisions can never be made in a confidential manner. Ethical challenges concerning resource allocation and access to health care is an area of growing conflict for rural physicians (Christianson 1998; Cook, Hoas, and Guttmannova 2002; Moscovice and Rosenblatt 2000; Schank 1998), nurses (Cook, Hoas, and Joyner 2000; Turner, Marquis, and Burman 1996), and administrators (Nelson 2004; see chap. 4).

Case 4 shows how disease stigma might present a significant ethical conflict because of the "fishbowl" nature of life in rural settings (Roberts, Battaglia, and Epstein 1999). Close-knit rural communities can spur ethical conflicts, particularly those involving mental health care because of its related stigma and interpersonal complexity (Campbell and Gordon 2003; Roberts and Dyer 2004; see chap. 7). As the patient in Case 4 notes, everyone will recognize his truck parked at the mental health professional's office. Rural residents may be uncomfortable with the prospect of disclosing information to the health care provider or may not seek the necessary care (Henderson 2000; Jennings 1992; Spiegel 1990), resulting in mental health disorders that go undiagnosed and untreated while compromising the quality of care and the provider-patient relationship (Roberts et al. 1999; Roberts and Dyer 2004). Rural health care professionals may be more reluctant than their urban counterparts to include a potentially stigmatizing diagnosis—such as HIV, mental illness, or a sexually transmitted infection—in a patient's medical record. This exclusion can also be requested, or demanded, by patients.

Overlapping relationships, as illustrated in Case 5, can lead to conflicts of interest that are unknown in nonrural settings. The physician recognizes that her fiduciary responsibility to the patient requires her to primarily be a patient advocate, to promote the health and well-being of her patient and the fetus. However, the lack of other options for childcare complicates the decision to recommend bed rest for her patient. The physician must balance the patient's needs, her own needs as a mother, and the needs of others in the community who rely on her for health care.

The general ethical domains of boundary conflicts, disease stigma, access to health care, and conflicts of interest illustrated in these cases are familiar to all health care professionals. The cases underscore that rural health care issues cannot be separated from the rural environment and that the ethical conflicts faced rarely emphasize situations involving advanced medical technology.

Ethics Resources in Rural Settings

Despite the extent of ethical conflicts arising in rural health care, ethics resources that take into consideration the characteristics of rural settings are limited and, presumably, inadequate (see chap. 4). The ethics literature scarcely addresses rural issues, and there are few bioethicists in rural communities. Concerns about the adequacies of ethics committees in small rural hospitals have been expressed. Rural clinicians have commented that professional codes of ethics and guidelines are inattentive to the conflicts that exist in small communities (Roberts et al. 1999; Roberts and Dyer 2004). Furthermore, ethics training has such an urban bias that it provides little assistance to rural practitioners (Roberts et al. 1999; see chap. 12).

Limited Literature on Rural Ethics

A recent literature review found only 55 articles published between 1966 and 2004 to have specifically and substantively addressed rural health care ethics (Nelson et al. 2006). The authors found only seven original research articles that included formal research methods, 12 articles that provided descriptive summaries of research findings without a description of study methodologies, and 36 general commentaries or case studies. More than half (55%) of these publications examined clinical ethical conflicts, while 27 percent addressed organizational ethics and 18 percent addressed the ethical ramifications of rural health care policies at a national or community level. Most of these research publications used survey methods, had a small sample, and/or focused on a particular group of professionals, such as physicians, nurses, or hospital administrators; they also lacked urban-rural comparisons.

Limited Rural Bioethicists

Relatively few bioethicists work or live in rural U.S. communities, as evidenced by the geographic distribution of the 2004 membership of the

American Society for Bioethics and Humanities (ASBH) across the rural-urban continuum described at the beginning of the chapter (Nelson and Weeks 2006). Although 91 percent of ASBH members lived or worked in urban settings, only 2 percent lived or worked in rural settings. Furthermore, the rate of ASBH members to hospital facilities was one to three in urban areas and 1 to 100 in rural areas; more dramatic was the rate of members to hospital beds of 1 to 780 in urban areas and 1 to 5,360 in rural areas. Although not all bioethicists are ASBH members, these findings suggest that the availability of professional bioethical resources might be inadequate in the rural United States.

Ethics Committees

Ethics committees have a long history of working to improve the quality of health care by providing a forum to address ethical issues with a multidisciplinary group of health care professionals who have knowledge and skills in applied ethics. The traditional ethics committee has a generally accepted purpose, structure, and set of functions (Cranford and Doudera 1984; Lo 2000; Milmore 2006). The basic functions include ethics education, institutional policy review and development, and case consultation. Even though ethics committees vary in effectiveness, competency, structure, and function, they tend to have multidisciplinary professional members, a defined set of functions and processes, regular meetings, active members, clinical case consultation services, committee and staff ethics education, and a trained ethics expert available to advise and/or educate members (Aulisio, Arnold, and Youngner 2000; Hosford 1986; Jonsen 1998; Lo 2000; Milmore 2006; Nelson 2006).

Fewer small, rural health care facilities have ethics committees than do urban facilities. In a survey of 117 hospital administrators from six western states, only 42 percent of the hospitals had ethics committees (Cook, Hoas, and Guttmannova 2000). Only 16 percent of small hospitals, those with 25 beds or less, had ethics committees. The Joint Commission on the Accreditation of Healthcare Organizations (JCAHO) requires that hospitals have a "mechanism" to address ethics conflicts (2004). Not surprisingly, this study found that "small hospitals were less likely to have bioethics committees (R = 0.304, p < .01) and less likely to hold the . . . [JCAHO] accreditation (R = 0.365, p < .01)" (Cook, Hoas, and Guttmannova 2000). Nonrural hospitals were more likely to have JCAHO accreditation status

(Baldwin et al. 2004; Brasure, Stensland, and Wellever 2000; Chen et al. 2003).

In contrast, a more recent study of 116 hospitals in upstate New York conducted in 2001 found that 92 percent of all hospitals had ethics committees. Based on self-reported identification of hospital location as rural, suburban, or urban (41%, 29%, and 30%, respectively), ethics committees were reported to exist in the vast majority of hospitals irrespective of geographic location (rural 90%, suburban 89%, and urban 100%) (Milmore 2006). Similarly, another survey of 388 members of the American College of Healthcare Executives who were hospital CEOs from across the United States reported that 84 percent of their facilities had ethics committees (Ethics practices and beliefs 2006). In a more recent article, among 519 U.S. hospitals surveyed, 95 percent either had an ethics consultation service or were developing one (Fox, Myers, and Pearlman 2007). Despite the inconsistency among the various studies, there appear to be fewer ethics committees in rural hospitals than in urban hospitals.

For rural facilities that do have ethics committees, there can be many obstacles that undermine their effectiveness (see chaps. 3 and 9). These obstacles could include the lack of a professionally diversified membership, members' competing commitments, the inability to meet regularly, and the unavailability of adequate ethics training. Small rural hospitals tend to have a limited array of health care professionals, thereby reducing the possibility of having multidisciplinary members serve on their ethics committee (Nelson 2006). Professionals working at a rural facility also tend to have multiple professional responsibilities and may find serving on an ethics committee a significant burden in terms of time and travel. For example, imagine an ethics committee at a 36-bed rural hospital, chaired by a nurse administrator who also functions as the facility's compliance officer, patient safety officer, and quality improvement officer. Another committee member, a family physician, has to travel on challenging roads eighteen miles to the hospital from where his private practice is located to attend infrequent meetings. While it is true that professionals in large urban facilities may also have multiple responsibilities, small rural hospitals tend to have a limited number of professionals on their staffs so these problems are exacerbated.

Based on my experience and a recent study (Milmore 2006), most traditional ethics committees meet bimonthly or monthly, whereas such regular meetings at rural facilities may not occur. One study reported that only

10 percent of facilities had ethics committees that met regularly (Cook, Hoas, and Guttmannova 2000). Opportunities to meet regularly can be limited as a result of members' availability and competing duties.

Adequate ethics training for committee members is essential. In general, many committees in U.S. hospitals have a limited number of members with formal ethics training (Fox, Myers, and Pearlman 2007; Milmore 2006). However, rural ethics committee chairs and members may lack not only adequate training but also pertinent ethics resources. Consider the challenges encountered by the family physician member of that 36-bed hospital ethics committee who might want to attend an ethics seminar. The physician will have to find an ethics training that addresses rural-focused issues. If the physician is able to do so, he will have to try to find financial resources to cover traveling expenses from a rural health care facility's limited budget. Additionally, the physician will have to arrange medical coverage from a colleague in another town, with the understanding that coverage will be provided for that physician when needed. The physician must also accept the reality of lost revenue. The list of challenges is extensive.

As a result, few rural ethics committee members or others who provide ethics case consultation appear to possess even the basic core competencies to perform ethics case consultations as recommended by the Core Competency for Health Care Ethics Consultation (Arnold 1998; Aulisio, Arnold, and Youngner 2000). These competencies cover nine areas of knowledge, 12 skills areas, and several important personal characteristics. The report recommended that committee members performing case consultations should possess a basic level of the identified knowledge and skills (Arnold 1998; Aulisio, Arnold, and Youngner 2000). A survey of West Virginia rural bioethics network members noted that the members felt they possessed less than the basic level in several of the knowledge and skills areas needed to address common ethical conflicts (Moss 1999). The survey also noted that respondents did not possess the advanced level of knowledge to consult on the most complex cases.

Rural health care providers share the need for relevant ethics resources. A survey of nurses indicated the lack of ethics-related resources was a major concern. Seventy-two percent of the nurses believe ethics-related resources are necessary in rural health care settings, and more than 88 percent specifically requested resources that address professional responsibilities (Cook and Hoas 2000; Cook, Hoas, and Joyner 2000). Preliminary analysis of a recent survey of primary care providers and hospital administrators in rural New England indicates a strong need for a variety of rural-focused resources, including effective ethics committees (Nelson et al. 2007).

The need for effective rural ethics committees begs the question: How should rural health care facilities respond to the need for competent and effective ethics committees? One possible approach is to develop and implement strategies at the local hospital to systemically identify and overcome barriers that hamper efforts to create and maintain an effective ethics committee (Niemira 1988). Ethics expertise can be developed through ongoing, independent study and, possibly, attendance at seminars. Once the ethics expert has attained an appropriate level of expertise, he or she would provide ethics training to the other committee members. The increased competency could expand the committee's role to include case consultation and policy development (Niemira 1988; Niemira, Orr, and Culver 1989). This strategy may prove effective at facilities where there is institutional support and an identified ethics leader willing to pursue such training and able to nurture the other committee members.

Local ethics committee members may also be able to receive training to create an ongoing linkage with a state's ethics network (Rauh and Bushy 1990). However, a few rural states—West Virginia, Maine (see chap. 9), New Mexico, New Hampshire, and Vermont—have established such networks. As several ethics committee members have poignantly indicated to me after attending nonrural network training programs, they felt out of place at such meetings because network leaders, presenters, and the majority of participants were from large urban academic facilities and were unfamiliar with the particulars of rural health care issues.

Another response to the need for competent and effective ethics resources at rural hospitals is to consider the possibility that the traditional model for ethics committees is not useful to a small, isolated, rural health care facility (Nelson 2006; Niemira, Meece, and Reiquam 1989). Building on earlier proposals for ethics committees in rural settings (Cook, Hoas, and Guttmannova 2000; Niemira, Meece, and Reiquam 1989; Rauh and Bushy 1990) is the implementation of the multifacility ethics committee (MFEC) (Nelson 2006).

The MFEC approach, as previously presented in greater detail (Nelson 2006), provides several of the basic functions of the traditional model while potentially overcoming many of the obstacles that limit the effectiveness of rural local ethics committees. A multifacility approach would link the ethics talent from several facilities. The model is particularly feasible where there are existing networks of facilities or a multisite health system. The MFEC would allow facilities to share education resources, ethics expertise, and financial support as well as reduce duplication of efforts.

As suggested, each facility participating in the MFEC would identify one or two committee members to serve on the regional or network-based committee. Even for members who lack ethics training, the primary criteria for selection would be a willingness to participate in the meetings, a desire to develop ethics knowledge and skills, and some available time. "Each participating facility would provide financial support for its representative(s) and modest support for MFEC's general operation. The financial support could be pooled without overly taxing any individual facility. Because the geographical distances between facilities can be significant, regular meetings could be conducted by telephone conference calling or where available video-teleconferencing" (Nelson 2006, p. 194).

The overall purpose of the MFEC would be to foster ethical practices at member facilities through two primary functions: ethics education and the proactive development and propagation of ethical guidelines to address recurring ethics issues. First, because there is a lack of local ethics expertise at rural facilities (Cook and Hoas 2000; Niemira, Orr, and Culver 1989; Roberts et al. 1999), education activities should seek to promote the knowledge and skills of MFEC members to respond to rural ethics conflicts and to support efforts to facilitate ethics education at the local facility. Second, committees should shift from reacting to ethics conflicts on a case-by-case basis to trying to reduce the occurrence of common ethical conflicts by proactively developing ethical practice guidelines. The MFEC would address recurring conflicts that beg for ethical guidelines to assist the clinician in response to the conflict. It is a proactive, preventive, systems-oriented approach to health care ethics suggested by several authors (Chervenak and McCullough 2004; Forrow, Arnold, and Parker 1993; McCullough 1998, 2005; Nelson 2007). After the MFEC prepares ethical guidelines to address issues such as conflicts of interest or provider-patient boundary issues, the document would be shared with the local facility for review and potential implementation. Such a process could promote consistent and reasoned thinking while not burdening any one facility.

This untested MFEC model would need to be carefully planned, implemented, and assessed to determine its effectiveness in helping clinical and administrative staff respond to ethical conflicts. Such a model might be a more viable option where facilities have some level of connection, local ethics committees do not exist or are struggling, and facilities can provide administrative support.

The traditional model for ethics committees is well established but continues to evolve. Small, rural health care facilities have fewer ethics committees than their large, urban counterparts, despite the universal need for committees or resources to assist clinicians and administrators in addressing ethical conflicts. Even where facility administrators and/or clinicians recognize the importance of such committees, they are significantly challenged by lack of available ethics expertise, budget support, and an effective model for structuring the rural ethics committee (Cook and Hoas 1999; Nelson and Pomerantz 1992a; Niemira 1988; Niemira, Meece, and Reiquam 1989). Overcoming these obstacles to creating a traditional ethics committee in the rural setting is difficult because many of them are related to the characteristics of a rural health care facility. Therefore, rural health care facilities need to begin to develop, implement, and assess new models or approaches to "doing ethics."

Strategies for Addressing Rural Health Care Ethics

Health care professionals respond to ethical challenges occurring regularly within their clinical practices based on personal beliefs, experiences and training, community values, and their own interpretations of ethical guidelines. Because patients' quality of care can be influenced by the clinician's responses to the ethical challenges (see chap. 8), there is a need to explore practical strategies for addressing ethical conflicts. Therefore, several strategies are offered to address rural health care ethics; these practical strategies, some of which have previously been delineated (Nelson and Schmidek 2008), are intended for rural health care professionals (see chap. 3), rural health care organizations, state or regional ethics networks (see chap. 9), professionals' organizations, health care educators (see chap. 12), and health care ethicists:

- Rural health care professionals should seek to acquire a basic understanding of health care ethics, including an awareness of basic ethical standards of practice. Ethical standards are generally accepted guidelines for responding to common ethical conflicts. Even though these guidelines may lack a rural focus, they provide an important foundation from which to identify and to respond to ethical challenges. Ethical standards can be found in a wide variety of sources, including the American Medical Association's Ethics Manual (Kitchens et al. 1998; Lo 2000).

- Rural health care professionals should seek to develop a network of rural colleagues to be consulted to provide support or advice regarding ethical challenges. Seeking the perspective from other rural clinicians outside the immediate clinical situation might provide insight, clarity, and supportive advice. Colleagues also can discuss the ethical conflict with an intimate understanding of the rural culture (Roberts et al. 1999).
- Rural health care professionals should identify health care ethicists to provide consultation and training. Bioethicists might be available through the telephone, Internet, tele-health programs, and rural networks. Most academic-based ethics centers have Web sites that can provide ethics resources. Contact with ethicists as with clinician colleagues can alleviate a sense of isolation.
- Rural health care professionals should identify rural health care facilities with an ethics program or committee. They should learn who chairs the committee and how a provider can contact the committee to address an ethics question. The ethics committees at rural facilities may provide case consultation and education programs.
- Rural health care professionals should collaborate with a network of clinicians, ethicists, and ethics committee members to proactively draft and disseminate ethics practice guidelines for recurring rural ethical conflicts. The ethical conflicts raised in the previously described cases suggest the need to explore each of the conflicts and develop ethical practice guidelines. The ethical conflicts identified by the formal or informal network can be discussed to establish a general understanding of the best approach to respond to these conflicts. The process may seem arduous; however, the effort can diminish future conflicts, thus reducing time-consuming and stressful challenges (Chervenak and McCullough 2004; Forrow, Arnold, and Parker 1993; McCullough 1998, 2005; Nelson 2007).
- Rural health care professionals can provide local community-wide education programs on health care ethics issues, such as end-of-life

decision making or privacy and confidentiality, to foster community understanding. Such education events can be facilitated in collaboration with community leaders, such as clergy.

- Rural health care professionals can develop pamphlets delineating their ethical standards of practice to complement discussions with patients. The pamphlets can be available in waiting rooms. Proactive activities similar to community-wide education can enhance community understanding and foster a preventative ethics approach.
- Rural health care professionals can encourage health care conference planners at state or national professional meetings to include a focus on rural ethics issues. Meetings can provide an avenue to engage with others concerning rural health care, including ethical challenges.
- Rural health care professionals can actively participate and/or encourage national professional organizations to establish standards of care that include a rural perspective (see chap. 7).

In addition to rural health care professionals employing practical strategies, health care ethicists should implement strategies to address rural health care ethics issues that support the efforts of professionals in addressing ethical challenges (Nelson et al. 2007):

- Health care ethicists should increase their awareness and understanding of rural health care issues as perceived by residents and health care professionals, including the contextual influence on ethical issues and how the issues are different from those in nonrural settings.
- Health care ethicists should collaborate with rural health care professionals in drafting ethical guidelines for addressing common, recurring conflicts.
- Health care ethicists should develop and implement ethics training curricula and other educational resources for future nurses, clinicians, and administrators.
- Health care ethicists who serve as conference planners should include presentations and discussions of rural health care ethics issues at national or regional ethics meetings.
- Health care ethicists should expand their focus to include rural issues in the literature. Health care ethicists in collaboration with researchers should conduct or facilitate quantitative and qualitative

research to better understand rural health care ethics (Nelson et al. 2007).

Implications for Ethical Practices

Rural health care ethics is one of the subject areas of the broad discipline of health care ethics. Unfortunately, it has received less attention than other areas of focus of health care ethics, even though roughly 21 to 23 percent of the population lives in those areas (Institute of Medicine 2005; Nelson et al. 2007; Ricketts 2000; Roberts, Battaglia, and Epstein 1999).

What makes rural health care ethics special is how the rural environment influences ethical conflicts in the delivery of health care. Many rural residents have significant illness and injury-related disabilities, and they encounter tremendous obstacles when seeking needed health care. Rural Americans have limited access to clinicians, health facilities, and specialized services, and their care is hampered by geographic and climatic barriers, as well as heightened social, cultural, and economic challenges. Indeed, the burden of illness for rural populations is considerable, placing great demands on a resource-poor clinical care system. Consequently, rural people are increasingly recognized as an underserved, vulnerable population. An appropriate standard of care for rural people, moreover, has emerged as a concern in the national discussion of health disparities.

With the growth of interest in rural health care, an emerging awareness of the special ethical considerations inherent to clinical practice in closely knit, tightly interdependent small community settings has also begun to take place.

Despite the unique character of these emerging rural ethics issues, there are limited resources specifically focused to assist rural clinicians who are confronted with complex ethical dilemmas. For these reasons, we have identified several strategies for health care professionals and ethicists to address the need for fostering the work of rural health care ethics.

In the midst of these concerns, health care professionals who live and work in rural communities can and do experience wonderful, fruitful opportunities for in-depth, long-term patient relationships. As Megan Wills Kullnat writes, "Patients praise their physicians with loyalty that has become rare in medicine" (Kullnat 2007, p. 344). This rewarding experience led Michael J. Fox's character to give up his plan to practice plastic surgery in Beverly Hills for a life practicing family medicine in rural Grady, North Carolina. Many real-life health care professionals choose a similar path.

NOTES

I gratefully acknowledge the editing and research contributions of Jared M. Schmidek and Bette-Jane Crigger in the preparation of this chapter.

Funding for the preparation of this chapter comes from the White River Junction, Vermont VAMC Veteran's Rural Health Initiative and under an agreement with the State of New Hampshire, Department of Health and Human Services, Division of Public Health Services, with funds provided in part or in whole by the United States Department of Health and Human Services.

The views expressed in this chapter do not necessarily represent the views of the U.S. government.

REFERENCES

Arnold, R. M. 1998. *Core competencies for health care consultation.* Glenview, IL: American Society for Bioethics and Humanities.

Aulisio, M. P., R. M. Arnold, and S. J. Youngner. 2000. Health care ethics consultation: Nature, goals, and competencies. A position paper from the Society for Health and Human Values-Society for Bioethics Consultation Task Force on Standards for Bioethics Consultation. *Annals of Internal Medicine* 133 (1): 59–69.

Baldwin, L. M., R. F. MacLehose, L. G. Hart, S. K. Beaver, N. Every, and L. Chan. 2004. Quality of care for acute myocardial infarction in rural and urban U.S. hospitals. *Journal of Rural Health* 20 (2): 99–108.

Brasure, M., J. Stensland, and A. Wellever. 2000. Quality oversight: Why are rural hospitals less likely to be JCAHO accredited? *Journal of Rural Health* 16 (4): 324–36.

Bushy, A. 1993. Defining "rural" before tackling access issues. *American Nurse* 25 (8): 20.

———. 1994. When your client lives in a rural area. Part I: Rural health care delivery issues. *Issues in Mental Health Nursing* 15 (3): 253–66.

Butler, M. A., and C. L. Beale. 1994. *Rural-urban continuum codes for metro and nonmetro counties, 1993.* Washington, DC: U.S. Department of Agriculture.

Callahan, D. 1995. Bioethics. In *Encyclopedia of bioethics,* edited by W. T. Reich. New York: Simon & Schuster Macmillan.

Campbell, C. D., and M. C. Gordon. 2003. Acknowledging the inevitable: Understanding multiple relationships in rural practice. *Professional Psychology: Research and Practice* 34 (4): 430–34.

Chen, J., S. S. Rathore, M. J. Radford, and H. M. Krumholz. 2003. JCAHO accreditation and quality of care for acute myocardial infarction. *Health Affairs (Millwood)* 22 (2): 243–54.

Chervenak, F. A., and L. B. McCullough. 2004. An ethical framework for identifying, preventing, and managing conflicts confronting leaders of academic health centers. *Academic Medicine* 79 (11): 1056–61.

Christianson, J. 1998. Potential effects of managed care organizations in rural communities: A framework. *Journal of Rural Health* 14 (3): 169–79.

Cook, A., and H. Hoas. 1999. Are healthcare ethics committees necessary in rural hospitals? *HEC Forum* 11 (2): 134–39.

Cook, A. F., and H. Hoas. 2000. Where the rubber hits the road: Implications for organizational and clinical ethics in rural healthcare settings. *HEC Forum* 12 (4): 331–40.

———. 2001. Voices from the margins: A context for developing bioethics-related resources in rural areas. *American Journal of Bioethics* 1 (4): W12.

Cook, A. F., H. Hoas, and K. Guttmannova. 2000. Bioethics activities in rural hospitals. *Cambridge Quarterly of Healthcare Ethics* 9 (2): 230–38.

———. 2002. Ethical issues faced by rural physicians. *San Diego Journal of Medicine* 55 (6): 221–24.

Cook, A. F., H. Hoas, and J. C. Joyner. 2000. Ethics and the rural nurse: A research study of problems, values, and needs. *Journal of Nursing Law* 7 (1): 41–53.

Cranford, R. E., and A. E. Doudera, eds. 1984. *Institutional ethics committees and health care decision making.* Ann Arbor, MI: Health Administration Press.

Ethics practices and beliefs. 2006. *Healthcare Executive* 21 (6):74–75.

Flex Monitoring Team. 2007. *CAH Information.* Universities of Minnesota, North Carolina at Chapel Hill, and Southern Maine 2006. www.flexmonitoring.org/cahlistRA.cgi. Accessed March 19, 2007.

Forrow, L., R. M. Arnold, and L. S. Parker. 1993. Preventive ethics: Expanding the horizons of clinical ethics. *Journal of Clinical Ethics* 4 (4): 287–94.

Fox, E., S. Myers, and R. A. Pearlman. 2007. Ethics consultation in United States hospitals: A national survey. *American Journal of Bioethics* 7 (2): 13–25.

Gamm, L. D., L. L. Hutchinson, B. J. Dabney, and A. M. Dorsey, eds. 2003. *Rural health people 2010: A companion document to healthy people 2010.* Vol. 1. College Station: Texas A&M University System Health Science Center, School of Rural Public Health, Southwest Rural Health Research Center.

Hardwig, J. 2006. Rural health care ethics: What assumptions and attitudes should drive the research? *American Journal of Bioethics* 6 (2): 53–54.

Henderson, C. B. 2000. Small-town psychiatry. *Psychiatric Services* 51 (2): 253–54.

Hosford, B. 1986. *Bioethics committees: The health care provider's guide.* Rockville, MD: Aspen Systems.

Institute of Medicine. 2005. *Quality through collaboration: The future of rural health*. Washington, DC: National Academies Press.

Jennings, F. L. 1992. Ethics of rural practice. *Psychotherapy in Private Practice* 10:85–104.

Johnson-Webb, K. D., L. D. Baer, and W. M. Gesler. 1997. What is rural? Issues and considerations. *Journal of Rural Health* 13 (3): 253–56.

Joint Commission on the Accreditation of Healthcare Organizations. 2004. *Section 1: Patient-focused functions: Ethics, rights, and responsibilities (RI), 2004 automated hospitals CAMH refreshed core: Standards, rationales, elements of performance, scoring*. Oakbrook Terrace, IL: Joint Commission on the Accreditation of Healthcare Organizations.

Jonsen, A. 1998. *The birth of bioethics*. New York: Oxford University Press.

Kitchens, L. W., T. A. Brennan, R. J. Carroll, C. L. Clagett, L. L. Dunn, K. V. Eden, J. Lynn, S. H. Miles, G. J. Povar, D. L. Schiedermayer, S. H. Thompson, J. A. Tulsky. 1988. Ethics manual. 4th ed. American College of Physicians. *Annals of Internal Medicine* 128 (7): 576–94.

Klugman, C. M. 2006. Haves and have nots. *American Journal of Bioethics* 6 (2): 63–64.

Kullnat, M. W. 2007. A piece of my mind. Boundaries. *Journal of the American Medical Association* 297 (4): 343–44.

Larson, L. 2001. How many hats are too many? *Trustee* 54 (2): 1, 6–10.

Lo, B. 2000. *Ethical dilemmas: A guide for clinicians*. 2d ed. Philadelphia: Lippincott, Williams & Wilkins.

McCullough, L. B. 1998. Preventive ethics, managed practice, and the hospital ethics committee as a resource for physician executives. *HEC Forum* 10 (2): 136–51.

———. 2005. Practicing preventive ethics—the keys to avoiding ethical conflicts in health care. *Physician Executive* 31 (2): 18–21.

Miller, P. J. 1994. Dual relationships in rural practice: A dilemma of ethics and culture. *Human Services in the Rural Environment* 18 (2): 4–7.

Milmore, D. 2006. Hospital ethics committees: A survey in Upstate New York. *HEC Forum* 18 (3): 222–44.

Moscovice, I., and R. Rosenblatt. 2000. Quality-of-care challenges for rural health. *Journal of Rural Health* 16 (2): 168–76.

Moss, A. H. 1999. The application of the Task Force report in rural and frontier settings. *Journal of Clinical Ethics* 10 (1): 42–48.

National Center for Health Statistics. 2001a. Figure 3: Population by age, region, and urbanization level: United States, 1998. In *Health, United States, 2001, with urban and rural health chartbook*. Washington, DC: U.S. Government Printing Office.

———. 2001b. Figure 11: Infant mortality rates by region and urbanization level: United States, 1996–98. Data tables on urban and rural health. In *Health, United States, 2001, with urban and rural health chartbook*. Washington, DC: U.S. Government Printing Office.

————. 2001c. Figure 19: Suicide rates among persons 15 years of age and over by sex, region, and urbanization level: United States, 1996–98. Data tables on urban and rural health. In *Health, United States, 2001, with urban and rural health chartbook*. Washington, DC: U.S. Government Printing Office.

Nelson, W. 2004. Addressing rural ethics issues. The characteristics of rural health-care settings pose unique ethical challenges. *Healthcare Executive* 19 (4): 36–37.

————. 2006. Where is the evidence: A need to assess rural ethics committee models. *Journal of Rural Health* 22 (3): 193–95.

Nelson, W., M. Goodrich, J. Weiss, and M. Lawrence. 2007. Frequency of Ethical Challenges for Primary Care Providers: A Pilot Study. Unpublished data.

Nelson, W., G. Lushkov, A. Pomerantz, and W. B. Weeks. 2006. Rural health care ethics: Is there a literature? *American Journal of Bioethics* 6 (2): 44–50.

Nelson, W., A. Pomerantz, K. Howard, and A. Bushy. 2007. A proposed rural healthcare ethics agenda. *Journal of Medical Ethics* 33 (3): 136–39.

Nelson, W., and W. B. Weeks. 2006. Rural and non-rural differences in membership of the American Society of Bioethics and Humanities. *Journal of Medical Ethics* 32 (7): 411–13.

Nelson, W. A. 2007. Decreasing ethical conflicts. *Healthcare Executive* 22:36–38.

Nelson, W. A., and A. S. Pomerantz. 1992a. Ethics issues in rural health care. *Trustee* 45 (8): 14–15.

————. 1992b. Ethics issues in rural health care. In *Choices and conflict: Explorations in health care ethics*, edited by E. Friedman. Chicago: American Hospital Publishers.

Nelson, W. A., and J. M. Schmidek. 2008. Rural Health Care Ethics. In *The Cambridge textbook for bioethics*, edited by P. A. Singer and A. M. Viens, pp. 289–98. New York: Cambridge University Press.

Niemira, D. A. 1988. Grassroots grappling: Ethics committees at rural hospitals. *Annals of Internal Medicine* 109 (12): 981–83.

Niemira, D. A., K. S. Meece, and C. W. Reiquam. 1989. Multi-institutional ethics committees. *HEC Forum* 1 (2): 77–81.

Niemira, D. A., R. D. Orr, and C. M. Culver. 1989. Ethics committees in small hospitals. *Journal of Rural Health* 5 (1): 19–32.

Purtilo, R., and J. Sorrell. 1986. The ethical dilemmas of a rural physician. *Hastings Center Report* 16 (4): 24–28.

Purtilo, R. B. 1987. Rural health care: The forgotten quarter of medical ethics. *Second Opinion* 6:10–33.

Rauh, J. R., and A. Bushy. 1990. Biomedical conflicts in the heartland. A system-wide ethics committee serves rural facilities. *Health Progress* 71 (2): 80–83.

Ricketts, T. C. 2000. The changing nature of rural health care. *Annual Review of Public Health* 21: 639–57.

Roberts, L. W., J. Battaglia, and R. S. Epstein. 1999. Frontier ethics: Mental health care needs and ethical dilemmas in rural communities. *Psychiatric Services* 50 (4): 497–503.

Roberts, L. W., J. Battaglia, M. Smithpeter, and R. S. Epstein. 1999. An office on Main Street: Health care dilemmas in small communities. *Hastings Center Report* 29 (4): 28–37.

Roberts, L. W., and A. R. Dyer. 2004. Caring for people in small communities. In *Concise guide to ethics in mental health care,* edited by L. W. Roberts and A R. Dyer. Washington, DC: American Psychiatric Publishing.

Rourke, L. L., and J. T. Rourke. 1998. Close friends as patients in rural practice. *Canadian Family Physician* 44:1208–10, 1219–22.

Schank, J. A. 1998. Ethical issues in rural counselling practice. *Canadian Journal of Counselling* 32 (4): 270–83.

Spiegel, P. B. 1990. Confidentiality endangered under some circumstances without special management. *Psychotherapy: Theory, Research, Practice Training* 27 (4): 636–43.

Turner, L. N., K. Marquis, and M. E. Burman. 1996. Rural nurse practitioners: Perceptions of ethical dilemmas. *Journal of the American Academy of Nurse Practitioners* 8 (6): 269–74.

U.S. Census Bureau. 1995. Urban and rural definitions. www.census.gov/population/censusdata/urdef.txt. (accessed March 19, 2007).

———. 2006. *United States Census 2000: Census 2000 urban and rural classification.* www.census.gov/geo/www/ua/ua_2k.html (accessed March 19, 2007).

Washington State Department of Health. 2006. Guidelines for using rural-urban classification systems for public health assessment. www.doh.wa.gov/Data/guidelines/RuralUrban.htm#4tier (accessed April 18, 2007).

Weeks, W. B., L. E. Kazis, Y. Shen, Z. Cong, X. S. Ren, D. Miller, A. Lee, and J. B. Perlin. 2004. Differences in health-related quality of life in rural and urban veterans. *American Journal of Public Health* 94 (10): 1762–67.

WWAMI Rural Health Research Center. 2006. Rural-urban commuting area codes (version 2.0). University of Washington. http://depts.washington.edu/uwruca/index.html (accessed March 19, 2007).

CHAPTER 3

Ethics, Errors, and Where We Go from Here

ANN FREEMAN COOK, PH.D., AND HELENA HOAS, PH.D.

Voices from the Margins

The director of nursing in the small rural hospital was willing to participate in a key informant interview. She questioned, however, what she could offer on the subject of ethics. Ethics, she explained, seemed like an academic pursuit, an area of study more suited to college classrooms than to rural hospitals. She acknowledged that ethical problems *could* develop in health care settings, noting—with some certainty—that a person who was a Jehovah's Witness could not receive blood transfusions. But overall, she did not think ethical problems occurred frequently in rural health care settings.

After talking for nearly an hour about the kinds of problem that did occur in her hospital, she noted that her personal values sometimes created dilemmas she could not easily resolve. She recounted several recent experiences: a physician who prescribed an outmoded treatment for wound care, a patient who suffered from the effects of a hematoma when appropriate diagnostic tests were not ordered, a young mother denied pain relief during childbirth because her husband and their religious community opposed it, and a patient who had inadvertently received an excessive dose of insulin. "These kinds of issues have occurred in our hospital," she noted. "They are not good for the patient. But are those *ethical* problems? I am not sure that I know what bioethics really is."

In this chapter we outline ethics issues commonly experienced by health care providers in rural areas, how they are handled, and the barriers that stand in the way of resolving them. To more fully explore the practical implications of our findings, we then examine ethical issues associated with provision of safe care, an ongoing challenge for rural hospitals. Finally, we discuss practical approaches that support recognition and resolution of ethical issues in rural health care settings.

Challenges to Ethics

It is important to understand that the nurse's questions about the scope of "ethics" are not unique. Similar perceptions, experiences, and uncertainties about what ethics really involves have surfaced in a series of multimethod studies among rural health care providers, patients, and community leaders in a multistate area (see chap. 5). These studies, conducted over a 10-year period and supported by the Culpeper/Rockefeller Brothers Fund, the Greenwall Foundation, and the Agency for Healthcare Research and Quality (AHRQ), used surveys, focus groups, key informant interviews, and textual analysis of responses to case studies to analyze what ethics-related issues occur and how they are recognized, discussed, reported, and resolved in rural health care settings.

As we have pursued these studies, we have frequently been asked to clarify the differences in the kinds of ethical problems that develop in rural versus urban settings. There may be no simple or straightforward response to that question. The rural bioethics literature offers a catalogue of conditions, such as confidentiality, familiarity, boundary issues, dual relationships, and resource scarcity that characterize the rural environment. While these conditions are certainly part of the rural environment, however, they do not constitute discrete, stand-alone ethical issues. For example, most rural health care providers frequently encounter issues associated with confidentiality but do not experience it as an ethical problem. Rather, they explained, they have learned how to deal with it. Similarly, most rural health care providers experience dual relationships but do not perceive such relationships as a burdensome ethical problem (see chaps. 2 and 7). They reported that knowing a patient and family helped them provide good care.

At any time, intervening factors, such as economic disparities (see chap. 4), can make a neutral condition into a problematic one. For example, a rural provider reported that the ER staff had caused a family great harm when they saved the life of a young boy who had been seriously injured in an accident. She noted that they took extreme measures because "they knew the boy and his family so well." The boy survived, although in an extremely disabled state. The economic consequences for the family have been severe. The family was forced to sell their farm land and other assets to pay for his rehabilitation. The emotional burdens have also been heavy; now that the child has returned home, his family must provide round-the-clock care. The health care provider feels guilty about the decisions made in the ER that day. She notes, "I see them around town almost every day." She explained that if she worked in an urban setting, she might not ever see the economic and emotional repercussions of the decisions made that day in the ER. But in a rural community the repercussions are clearly visible. She views the level of intervention that was provided in the ER as an abuse of power, a series of actions that served the interests of the health care team rather than the interests of the child and family.

In the case above, the child was known and well loved. As a result of this familiarity, heroic and perhaps even extreme measures were undertaken to save the child's life. In a different case, familiarity proved to be a factor that limited care. A poor family of low social standing needed a vaccination for a premature infant. The vaccination was expensive, and the family had no means to pay. Health care providers reported that the family had already received more than their fair share of health care services; the vaccination was not an emergency, and efforts to provide it would create a financial burden for the hospital. Both the health care providers and the family viewed the decision to deny care as one that involved distributive justice—but from different perspectives.

Similar stories about morally challenging bedside issues emerged in all the communities in which we conducted research. Rural health care providers, however, did not believe that ethics committees would help resolve such problems. Charles E. Rosenberg (1999) describes how ethics committees are viewed as focusing on the visible problematic instances rather than less dramatic policy debates and mundane bedside dilemmas. Thus, given the general beliefs about what ethics committees typically do, they were not viewed as particularly relevant, practical, or helpful in rural areas (Cook and Hoas 1999; Cook, Hoas, and Guttmannova 2000). "As far as I know," noted one rural administrator, "most ethics committees are dormant, floundering, or somewhere in between" (Cook and Hoas 1999, p. 134).

His assertion is supported by our survey data that indicate most rural hospitals lack ethics committees (Cook and Hoas 1999, 2000; Cook, Hoas, and Guttmannova 2000). Some ethics committees have been disbanded because they were too difficult to sustain. In cases where they did exist, few committees met the competencies required by such entities as the American Society for Bioethics and Humanities. Most of these committees met irregularly. In fact, only 10 percent of survey respondents reported that the committee in their hospital met on a regular basis. When committees did meet, the agendas appeared limited (see chaps. 2 and 9). Respondents noted that the committee's educational activities, for example, typically extended only to educating the members of the committee and rarely involved efforts to educate other staff members or patients. A minority— less than 30 percent—of existing committees reported any role in policy development, review, or evaluation, functions that are generally considered typical for ethics committee work in urban settings. Even fewer committees reported participation in case consultation, research, evaluation, or activities associated with patient advocacy. Among all possible functions, those associated with patient advocacy were provided least frequently (Cook, Hoas, and Guttmannova 2000).

Our data also suggest that the roles of ethics committee members may be rigidly defined. Physicians often have a leadership role. They convene meetings, determine agenda items, lead conversations, and delegate tasks. A rural nurse administrator offered the following representative comment: "We have a committee but it only meets twice a year. We don't review cases or develop policies. If we had to meet more often, the committee would probably disband" (Cook and Hoas 2000, p. 332). This comment reflects the fact that rural health care providers wear many hats; they serve on multiple committees and fulfill multiple roles. A nurse manager working in a rural hospital explained: "I'm everything, the director of nursing for the hospital and the nursing home, quality control manager, community liaison, safety officer, equal opportunity officer and just about anything and everything in between" (Cook, Hoas, and Joyner 2000, p. 43).

These demanding working conditions make rural health care providers unlikely to take part in an activity that is not deemed absolutely essential or helpful. Indeed, one of our studies found that more than 75 percent of physicians and 93 percent of nurses had never served on an ethics committee at any time during their training or professional careers (Cook and Hoas 2001; Cook, Hoas, and Guttmannova 2002). And regardless of whether health care providers had access to an ethics committee, there was no appreciable difference in the percentage of health care providers who sought their advice; the vast majority of physicians (75%) and nurses (93%) reported they had never referred a case to an ethics committee at any time in their careers.

When asked to describe what ethics-related resources they did use, physicians consistently noted their reliance on personal values and personal experiences. They identified as resources their spouses, the Ten Commandments, peers, or a close friend. Nurses also indicated a reliance on personal values and noted that they talked to peers or "took problems home." In part, there is such a reliance on informal systems because people in rural communities are aware of the web of connections between hospital staff and patients and are hesitant to take actions that may overtly jeopardize relationships. The use of a formal structure elevates an issue to a more prominent and perhaps more adversarial level.

Because of the interrelated factors that influence decision making in rural communities—relationships, resources, skills, working conditions, job security—a great deal is at stake. These interrelated factors may explain our finding that rural health care providers are unlikely to take action unless three conditions are met: shared recognition of a problem, belief that the consequences of recognition/action can be handled, and belief that something will change if one takes action. Repeatedly, we found that if one of these conditions was not met, the willingness to take action diminished and the three-legged milk stool toppled.

This theoretical construct helps explain what happens in rural settings, why some issues are resolved and some persistently ignored. It helps explain responses to more individual ethics-related problems. For example, the health care providers chose not to offer pain relief during childbirth because they did not want to contribute to potentially devastating reactions from a church's congregation. A nurse chose not to question a doctor's outmoded and problematic treatment of wound care because doing so would result in unmanageable personal consequences such as reassignment of duties, a reprimand, or long-term hostility from a member of the small medical staff.

Challenges to Safe Health Care

This milk stool construct also explains why it is so difficult to resolve system-level issues that create ethical complications. The chronic challenge of ensuring safe health care serves as an example of a system-level problem. Certainly the failure to deliver safe health care can raise a number of issues that have ethical implications. The adage "do no harm" is endorsed in both medical and nonmedical circles. The disclosure of error involves issues associated with autonomy, truth telling, evasion, and denial. Compensation for error involves issues associated with justice, allocation, and access to care. But if health care providers do not believe that there is agreement about what constitutes an error, that they can handle consequences such as reporting or disclosure, and that change will probably occur, adoption of safe practices is undermined.

The linkage between ethics and error has not been extensively explored in the bioethics literature. To explore this intersection we conducted nine studies during a four-year period among physicians, nurses, pharmacists, and administrators who work in rural hospitals in a nine-state area of the West. The methodology, including surveys, interviews, questionnaires, and textual analysis of responses to case studies, provided a way to examine cognitive, behavioral, and organizational constraints that influence recognition and resolution of ethical issues associated with patient safety (Cook et al. 2004). This approach provided a way to incorporate conceptual and empirical perspectives that influence our understanding of ethics in rural areas.

Our survey data show that most rural health care providers believe that they and their hospitals are genuinely concerned about patient safety. When asked to rate their ability to make health care safer, respondents to a staff survey of providers gave themselves high scores, a median and mode of 8 on a 10-point scale. Most endorsed, on system and individual levels, the "no shame / no blame" approach to errors that has been promulgated by the Institute of Medicine. Most health care providers said they want to learn about errors so they do not repeat mistakes. Finally, most (65%) said they feel comfortable discussing the topic of medical errors (Cook et al. 2004).

While these findings are encouraging, the aggregation of our data from all of the studies indicates that rural health care providers consistently demonstrate discrepancies in their abilities to recognize errors, report errors, allocate responsibility for patient safety, design interventions that increase patient safety, implement new practices, and sustain change (Cook and Hoas 2004). Moreover, among the health care disciplines, there are vastly different perceptions as to what constitutes an error, who is a member of the patient care decision-making team, who holds responsibility for patient safety, if errors should be reported or disclosed, and how errors should be resolved or prevented. These findings suggest that, in spite of good intentions, it may prove difficult to adopt new interventions and simultaneously keep the milk stool balanced (Cook, Hoas, and Guttmannova 2005).

For example, when health care providers completed surveys that assessed the kinds of errors they actually reported and their experiences associated with those reports, a narrow repository of errors emerged. Health care providers primarily recognized and reported only three kinds of problems: medication-related errors (incorrect dose, time, or port), patient falls, and illegible handwriting. Problems associated with medication-related errors and patient falls often involve nursing, and indeed most health care providers ascribed primary responsibility for ensuring patient safety to nurses. In fact, only 22 percent of health care providers believed that responsibility for ensuring patient safety was evenly shared among the professions (Cook et al. 2004). When explaining this belief, one physician asserted: "Patient safety is an important issue but it's not my role" (Cook et al. 2005, p. 387).

When health care providers were given biweekly case studies and scenarios embedded with errors related to diagnosis and/or treatment, most health care providers were hesitant to acknowledge that an "error" had occurred. Even when the case study included the definitions of error developed by the Institute of Medicine (delays in treatment, use of outmoded treatments, failure to employ needed tests, failure to act on results of testing, errors in diagnosis and administration of treatment, or failure to communicate), health care providers still questioned whether an error had occurred. Physicians, for example, generally viewed the errors contained in the case studies as "practice variances," "suboptimal outcomes," or examples of differences in "clinical judgment." Because physicians indicated an error *had not* occurred, they generally deemed specific interventions such as disclosure to the patient, notations in the chart, referral to hospital-based Morbidity and Mortality (M&M) meetings, compensation, or filing of incident reports as unnecessary and inappropriate. Physicians also expressed hesitancy to talk to one another about errors. As one respondent explained during an interview: "We just don't talk about that [error] stuff with one another."

Nurses who analyzed the case studies were also hesitant to designate treatment and diagnostic problems as errors, noting that they lacked the authority and the collegiality to question a physician's decisions. Indeed, nurses reported they were not encouraged to question orders or clinical decisions. "The doctor told me this was not an error," explained one typical respondent. Another noted: "The doctor said, 'So now you think you're licensed to practice medicine?'" Still another noted: "I have questioned his decisions and now he [the doctor] refuses to talk to me." And another: "You don't do things that may make a doctor decide to leave the hospital." Nurses noted that questionable situations may be referred to the hospital's M&M committee, but results of the deliberation may not be disclosed. Finally, nurses also reported poor access to resources such as authoritative clinical guidelines, pathways, standards of practice, and alerts when standards change. Without access to reliable resources, they lacked the confidence, knowledge, training, and authority to question unsafe clinical practices (Cook et al. 2004).

Administrators generally acknowledged their responsibility for ensuring patient safety in their institutions. However, they also noted that they lack the clinical knowledge to determine if certain clinical events should be deemed as errors and so defer to the judgment of physicians and M&M meetings (Cook et al. 2004). While this orientation is understandable, it compromises the ability of administrators to assume a leadership role in increasing patient safety in their hospitals. While pharmacists were more confident about their abilities to *recognize* certain kinds of errors—such as an incorrect dose or drug—they also noted that perceptions of their role inhibit their abilities to take action. Thus a pharmacist might characterize as "poor medical management" the care of a patient who is struggling with serious side effects caused by a treatment regimen involving 20 different medications, but corrective actions—such as a medication review—might not be pursued.

While most health care providers who participated in these studies claimed they were comfortable talking about errors, few had ever participated in *any* error resolution process, including investigation, review, or analysis of errors. Moreover, health care providers reported that they do not attend the same trainings, do not use the same resources and guides, rarely talk across disciplines, and have not developed strategies to identify or examine errors or mistakes associated with diagnosis and treatment. So there was not, they reported, much agreement about what constitutes an error, what guides to use, or what issues to report.

Implications for Ethical Practices

Our studies show that rural health care ethics is complex, subtle, and multidimensional, requiring a sophisticated understanding of the rural context. Issues that do not seem "ethical" when viewed through the traditional bioethics lens may have many ethical implications. It can be hard for health care providers to deal with these implications, and they are hesitant to take actions unless the milk stool conditions can be met. It is hard to say if the milk stool phenomenon is unique to rural communities or is present in the urban context as well.

Given the framework that has been traditionally used for bioethics, we do not know if the ethical problems that develop in rural areas are vastly different from those that develop in urban areas. We have learned, however, that the methodologies employed by the bioethics enterprise are not generally responsive to the kinds of problems that emerge in rural communities. Rural health care providers muddle through a maze of conflicting duties and responsibilities to arrive at good and fair decisions that reflect the norms and customs of their settings. In this milieu, the conventional stripped-down analytic models for ethical decision making are neither helpful nor useable.

We need to find new paradigms for framing issues and generating solutions. Given the large disparities among administrators, doctors, nurses, and pharmacists as to what constitutes an ethical issue, we are easily sidetracked and so ignore the moral issues that complicate everyday care. We may need to move from a philosophical analysis of discrete issues to one that allows a more sociological and anthropological examination of everyday patterns of care.

During the past 10 years, we have been working with interdisciplinary teams in our research hospitals to develop time-sensitive, collaborative approaches for resolving ethical dilemmas. Obviously, education is a critical component. But rural health care providers repeatedly noted a lack of time in their daily schedules for traditional educational activities. There was little interest in lengthy articles or academic lectures. There was little interest in the creation of new committees or consultation teams. Health care providers claimed they did not have time to log on to web sites and look for new information. And rural health care providers rarely had the time or the money to attend conferences and workshops.

We have found that one of the most successful educational strategies combines highly relevant case studies and e-mail (see chaps. 2 and 9). Short and succinct case studies that depict incidents that could or do occur in rural hospitals were e-mailed weekly to interdisciplinary teams of health care providers in participating hospitals. These cases provided a way to initiate and sustain dialogue. The health care providers were asked to analyze and respond to the cases by identifying issues, learning points, relevant guides, and specific strategies for improvement. By focusing on these kinds of practical issues, health care providers can figure out what they can realistically do to deliver ethical and safe health care.

The cases and responses were then shared with staff throughout the facilities in various ways; e-mail was used, but cases were also left on the nursing desks or posted in the lounges. Some hospitals hosted joint Continuing Medical Education (CME)/Continuing Education Units (CEU) meetings to discuss the cases. The case studies provided an accessible, recursive, collective learning opportunity that offered the same information, a safe forum for discussion, and a structure for envisioning and implementing new policies. "Before receiving these case studies," explained one nurse, "we never realized the extent to which we had totally different perceptions and definitions among professions. No wonder we didn't talk to one another."

These rural studies have provided useful information about the intersection between ethics and an ethics-related problem such as error. But additional multiple-method studies should be actively pursued so we can understand more completely the processes that support recognition of ethical issues, the belief that the consequences of recognition can be handled, and belief that change is possible. Such empirical knowledge will help us develop practical, inclusive, context-based approaches for enhancing ethical awareness on personal, professional, and organizational levels. New approaches could move the enterprise of ethics from the peripheral, sideline position of "something we don't have time for in rural areas" to a central bedside activity. Rural providers need to see ethics not as a luxury but as a necessity on which to build their practice.

REFERENCES

Cook, A., and H. Hoas. 1999. Are healthcare ethics committees necessary in rural hospitals? *HEC Forum* 11 (2): 134–39.

Cook, A., H. Hoas, and K. Guttmannova. 2005. From here to there: Lessons from an integrative patient safety project in rural healthcare settings. In *Advances in patient safety: From research to implementation,* edited by K. Henriksen, J. B. Battles, E. Marks, and D. I. Lewin. Washington, DC: Agency for Healthcare Research and Quality.

Cook, A. F., and H. Hoas. 2000. Where the rubber hits the road: Implications for organizational and clinical ethics in rural healthcare settings. *HEC Forum* 12 (4): 331–40.

———. 2001. Voices from the margins: A context for developing bioethics-related resources in rural areas. *American Journal of Bioethics* 1 (4): W12.

———. 2004. You have to see errors to fix them. *Modern Healthcare* 34 (49): 22.

Cook, A. F., H. Hoas, and K. Guttmannova. 2000. Bioethics activities in rural hospitals. *Cambridge Quarterly of Healthcare Ethics* 9 (2): 230–38.

———. 2002. Ethical issues faced by rural physicians. *San Diego Journal of Medicine* 55 (6): 221–24.

Cook, A. F., H. Hoas, K. Guttmannova, and J. C. Joyner. 2004. An error by any other name. *American Journal of Nursing* 104 (6): 32–43; quiz 44.

Cook, A. F., H. Hoas, and J. C. Joyner. 2000. Ethics and the rural nurse: A research study of problems, values, and needs. *Journal of Nursing Law* 7 (1): 41–53.

Rosenberg, C. 1999. Meanings, politics and medicine: On the bioethical enterprise and history. *Daedalus* 128 (4): 27–46.

CHAPTER 4

The Ethics of Allocating Resources toward Rural Health and Health Care

MARION DANIS, M.D.

Finding ways to distribute limited health care resources fairly and efficiently is among the most pivotal concerns in health care. The allocation of resources for the health of rural populations raises important questions regarding distributive justice and thus is the focus of this chapter. First, I review what makes rural populations vulnerable and difficult to care for with regard to their health. Then I explore the challenges to and opportunities for distributing resources effectively and equitably to rural populations. In the course of this chapter, I make use of the extensive literature on rural health and health care where it is pertinent.

The ethical analysis of resource allocation for rural health care proceeds in four steps: a brief characterization of rural health and health care, a consideration of the ethical implications of this characterization, an application of theories of distributive justice to priority setting for rural health care, and a consideration of the policy implications for rural health. I do not mean to imply that rural populations are necessarily always worse off than urban populations, which also pose challenges. However, the low density of rural populations poses some allocation issues that require solutions different from those that might work for urban populations.

Rural Health and Health Care

The extensive literature on rural health includes studies of the health behavior and status of rural populations (often but not always in comparison to urban populations), reports of the outcome of health services among rural populations, surveys of the manpower needs and the extent to which they are met, descriptions and evaluations of interventions intended to address the health care needs of rural communities, and reports of novel technological and organizational approaches to meeting the needs of rural populations. Literature about the status of the economy in rural areas and its effect on the well-being of rural residents is also pertinent. The literature indicates that many nations go to great lengths to address the health needs of their rural populations. Relevant aspects of this literature are reviewed here. While a large number of the studies mentioned here are from the United States, the intent of this review is to address issues of rural health and health care from an international perspective.

Rural Geography and Sociodemographics

Every region of the world has rural populations. Their ubiquitous presence means that while many rural areas are isolated, they share some common challenges with other rural populations. The United Nations Population Division (UNPD) does not have a uniform definition of rurality; rather, it uses those definitions assigned by nations themselves when reporting population statistics (United Nations Population Division 2005).[1] Furthermore, the definitions have been in flux. The United States currently designates areas with fewer than 2,500 persons as rural, whereas Canada and other Organization for Economic Cooperation and Development (OECD) countries use other definitions.[2]

To look at population trends, UNPD takes the newest definitions and applies them retrospectively. Every region of the world is experiencing a demographic shift in population from rural to urban areas. From 2010 to 2050, the world population is expected to go from 6.9 billion to 9.1 billion, but the rural population will go from 3.4 billion to 2.7 billion, thus dropping from 49.4 to 30.4 percent of world population (United Nations Population Division). By 2019, the absolute number of rural residents is expected to begin declining. The process of urbanization is uneven. In more developed regions of the world where 25.9 percent of the population lived in rural areas in 2005, 19.2 percent of the population will live in rural areas by 2030. In less developed regions taken as a whole (comprising all regions of Africa, Asia [including China but excluding Japan], Latin America and the Caribbean, Melanesia, Micronesia, and Polynesia), where

73.1 percent of the population lived in rural regions in 2005, the number is expected to diminish to 59.1 percent by 2030. When less developed regions of the world are examined in more detail, the rate of change appears varied as well. Latin America and the Caribbean are highly urbanized. Africa and Asia are less urbanized and are expected to experience more rapid shifts of population from rural to urban areas (United Nations Development Program 2005).

Thus, we can see that a crucial feature of many low-density populations is that they represent a steadily smaller percentage of the world's population. Yet the picture varies among rural communities. Some are more unstable than others. Formerly densely populated areas are losing population. This is the case, for example, in countries in Eastern Europe and the former Soviet bloc, which have undergone profound political change and have experienced massive population losses. As the population shifts from rural to urban areas, those who remain in rural areas are often further isolated and living in stagnant communities.

The economic picture that accompanies these demographic shifts is occasionally one of stark contrasts as rural and urban communities experience vastly uneven rates of development. In China, for instance, economic growth over the last twenty years has created a widening income gap. In 1985, Chinese rural peasants made half the income of urban residents, while in 2002 rural residents had only one-third of the income of urban residents (Weiping et al. 2006). Poverty has taken a marked toll on rural villages (Kahn and Yardley 2004).

Some of the most systematic data comparing rural and urban populations are available in the United States. The U.S. rural population is slightly older (with 18% enrolled in Medicare compared to 15% in urban areas) and has lower income (with an average per capita income of $19,000 compared to $26,000 among the urban population) than urban segments of the population. The extent to which this income difference translates into differences in poverty rates depends on the cost of living in rural and urban areas. A recent adjustment of poverty rates for geographic cost-of-living differences (using fair market rent to adjust for geographic differences) showed that the prevalence of poverty in nonmetropolitan areas is 12 percent less than in metropolitan areas of the United States (Joliffe 2006). Rural residents are also less likely to have private health insurance than the urban population (Rowley 2006; see also chaps. 1, 2, and 10).

If economic development bypasses rural areas, economic opportunities for rural populations are profoundly affected. The U.S. Department of Housing and Urban Development states, "In recent decades the United States rural economy has diversified, but economic stagnation and poverty remain problems in many rural communities. Many rural areas, given the lack of infrastructure and geographic isolation, are at a competitive disadvantage in the competition for jobs and industry" (2006). Aside from economic opportunities that bypass rural communities as the global economy grows, changes in the profile of the traditional rural economy also have a profound effect on economic prospects for rural residents. As farming has shifted from the family farm to agribusiness, agricultural employment opportunities for rural residents have diminished. In the United States, as of 2005, four out of five rural counties were dominated by non-farm activities such as mining, manufacturing, government operations, and tourism (Whitener 2005).

Epidemiology

Studies in the United States indicate that the health of rural populations is worse than that of urban populations by a variety of measures. These findings range along the spectrum from prevalence of health-risking behavior to morbidity and mortality. Rural adolescents have higher rates of smoking than adolescents in U.S. urban settings. Chronic diseases— hypertension (Huttlinger, Schaller-Ayers, and Lawson 2004) and diabetes (Andrus et al. 2004)—are less well controlled. Rural residents with acute problems also fare less well; trauma victims have higher mortality rates (Helling 2003). Studies of the health effects of disasters like earthquakes show that rural communities may be harder hit and less prepared than urban areas (Woersching and Snyder 2003; Helling 2003). The net result is that rural populations are known to have higher rates of premature mortality. The mortality rate for young (ages 1 to 24) rural males, for example, is 80 in 100,000 compared to 60 in 100,000 for urban males, and for young rural females is 40 in 100,000 compared to 30 in 100,000 for urban females (National Rural Health Association 2006).

Studies in Australia show parallel findings, with higher rates of death in rural communities, mainly due to coronary heart disease, other circulatory diseases, chronic obstructive pulmonary disease, motor vehicle accidents, diabetes, suicide, other injuries, and some cancers such as lung cancer. These higher death rates may relate to differences in access to services, risk factors, and the regional/remote environment (Australian Institute for Health and Welfare 2006).

Statistics from China show a life expectancy of 69.6 years for rural residents and 75.2 years for urban residents. Rural infant mortality is 34 percent in rural areas and 14 percent in urban areas (United Nations Development Program 2005).

The type of health problems existing in rural and urban populations may differ as a function of occupational differences. In the United States, osteoarthritis and undiagnosed joint pain are prevalent among rural agricultural workers: Osteoarthritis (10 to 12%) and back pain, joint injury, and orthopedic injury combined (38%) account for the major source of rural disability referrals (Kirkhorn, Greenlee, and Reeser 2003).

Any overview of the health status of a population must take into account socioeconomic factors, because level of education, income, and other social factors are important contributors to health (Marmot and Wilkinson 1999; WHO Commission on Social Determinants of Health 2005). To the extent that rural populations experience economic adversity, their health is likely to suffer. Studies of the relationship of socioeconomic determinants of health in rural areas show this correlation to be true (Kabir 2003; Sharma, Pradhan, and Padhi 2001; see also chap. 3).

Educational attainment tends to lag in rural communities, as demonstrated in the United States. While metropolitan areas had college completion rates of 26.6 percent, nonmetropolitan areas have completion rates of 15.5 percent as of 2000 (U.S. Department of Agriculture 2003). Rural residents who do not complete college are much more likely to be poor. Those without a high school degree had a poverty rate of 23.5 percent, whereas those with a college degree had a poverty rate of 3.5 percent. The degree of education of the work force also affects the likelihood of economic growth of a community. Nonmetropolitan areas with high school graduation rates below the average metropolitan rate lost 3.3 percent of their jobs in the 1990s, whereas those with high school graduation rates above the metropolitan average had an 8.7 percent gain in jobs (U.S. Department of Agriculture 2003).

Patterns of the Delivery and Organization of Health Care

In developed and developing countries, there is less access to medical personnel in rural areas. For example, in Canada, towns with fewer than

10,000 residents represent 22 percent of the population but have only 10 percent of the nation's physicians (Public Health Agency of Canada 2002). In India, 75 percent of the population lives in rural areas, but only 25 percent of that nation's physicians are located in them (Bagchi 2006).

A variety of adaptations have developed to deal with the health care needs of rural populations. To begin, rural residents often care for themselves to a great degree. Elders are often knowledgeable about sustaining health in austere conditions and caring for sick individuals using simple measures (Averill 2003). As a consequence, many patients self-medicate and often take over-the-counter and alternative medications (Vallerand, Fouladbakhsh, and Templin 2004). Large numbers of people also take one another's medications (Huttlinger, Schaller-Ayers, and Lawson 2004). But there is often a lack of health information and a proliferation of unhealthy behavior. For example, a rural sample of individuals in North Dakota was particularly uninformed about sun exposure. Only 18 percent wore sunscreen when anticipating sun exposure (Moore et al. 2003). In a report of rural Vietnamese knowledge about the likelihood of tuberculosis when experiencing a chronic cough, many did not realize the need to seek medical attention (Hoa et al. 2003). In their efforts to address their health needs, community-based action groups often work to decrease fragmentation of services (Averill 2003). How this behavior compares to urban populations is unclear, because these studies did not address urban populations.

Rural health care professionals are hard working and dedicated. A description of rural mental health nursing portrays a "relationship of intense professional intimacy and trust against a context of geographical disadvantage and professional isolation. The meanings of the relationship are elaborated in terms of unusually high levels of responsibility, professional ingenuity, powerlessness and the independent and risky character of life in the bush" (Gibb 2003, p. 243). Qualitative research indicates that rural practitioners find both positive and negative aspects to their work. In a survey in New Zealand, rural practitioners reported forming strong relationships with patients and community and enjoying the delivery of a wide spectrum of services. Negative features of their work included heavy workload, frequent on-call duties, lack of time off, and feeling undervalued and underpaid (Janes and Dowell 2004).

The intensity of the workload and commitment required by rural health care has implications for the character of the health care workforce. The profile of rural providers is heavily slanted toward nonphysician practitioners. This is true both for primary care (Grumbach et al. 2003) and specialty care providers. For example, in a study of the distribution of anesthesia providers, 8.4 percent of anesthesiologists were reported to reside in rural areas, but 18.6 percent of certified registered nurse anesthetists reside in nonmetropolitan areas (Fallacaro and Ruiz-Law 2004). Not surprisingly, retention of more highly trained practitioners is lower. In a study of length of stay for various practitioners in rural Alaska, health aides stayed an average of 1,186 days and doctors stayed 596 days; nurses stayed for the shortest length of time at 408 days.

At the organizational level, a variety of strategies have been developed to address the medical needs of rural populations. These include mobile clinics, as demonstrated by reports for treatment of dental and eye diseases (Labiris et al. 2003). In a study of specialty (oncology) clinics in Britain, three different organizational arrangements have been reported: central clinics, shared care outreach clinics with chemotherapy, and shared clinics without chemotherapy provision (Smith and Campbell 2004).

Some rural programs are particularly farsighted (see chap. 12). For example, an innovative model of home-based neonatal care in rural India involved trained female village health workers making repeated home visits during pregnancy and the neonatal period. Neonatal mortality decreased from 62 to 25 per 1,000 live births (Parker and Martin 2004). Some programs are based on a clear understanding that health status is a consequence of more than health services. For example, the Family Health and Rural Improvement Program in Papua New Guinea helped 300 families in twenty communities to acquire a water supply, sanitation, nutritional gardens, and small livestock and also provided health education. The program improved health and promoted development (Vail 2002).

The Use of Technology in Rural Health Care

The most farsighted practices in rural health have applied technology to overcome the barriers imposed by distance. Telemedicine has been used to increase access to services relatively cost-effectively, to improve health outcomes and quality of care, and to offer social support (Jennett et al. 2003). In a report on the use of telemedicine for treatment of pediatric diabetes and other endocrine problems, three modes were detailed: coordination of routine specialist clinics, ad hoc patient consultations for collaboration about acute and urgent problems, and delivery of education to rural staff (Smith et al. 2003).

Simple telephone practice is also found to be useful. A report from Australia described how a telepharmacy was designed with the intent of allowing community pharmacists to have real-time contact with dispensing doctors, aboriginal health workers, and patients in depot pharmacies (pharmacies without a pharmacist). While the study was designed to use videophones, video was not used because connection could not be established. The conventional phone served to address pharmacy needs, and the program was received enthusiastically. Use of the plain old telephone system (POTS) has been used for delivering cost-saving care by a school nurse who is linked to a mental health consultant, pediatric practitioner, and child psychiatrist (Young and Ireson 2003).

A striking example of applied technology is the use of geospatial information technology to tailor services to rural (and other vulnerable) populations (Faruque et al. 2003). By using geographic information systems, global positioning systems, and remote sensing, faculty members at the University of Mississippi were able to locate and collect information about rural residents, link this information to other health records, screen residents for health status, and develop and use a mobile clinic to treat and follow the population, with the aim of improving the collective health status of residents within a geographically defined area. This technique was used not only for clinical care but also for data gathering and research purposes to advance the field.

Common and Differing Themes across Rural Communities

In considering the features of rural health and health care, one should note the common and divergent features in order to consider what are valid generalizations that may be useful for ethical analysis. Some rural communities are poorer than others; some are more ethnically diverse or have an ethnic population that is more in the minority than other communities. The degree of isolation may also differ among communities, and the degree of rural isolation brings different clinical practice characteristics. The more rural or remote the area, the more likely a general practitioner is to be engaged in complete care (Humphreys et al. 2003). Whether a rural community is in a resource-poor or resource-rich area, or a developed or developing country, also influences its relative level of advantage or disadvantage. Another important consideration is that rural areas in developed countries are often pressed to recruit practitioners from other countries, but the consequences are often threatening to health care in resource-poor countries left behind by the practitioners (Drugger 2004; Ovrill and Stilwell 2004).

Characterization of Rurality in Ethical Terms

What might this summary of rural communities, their health status, and the character of their health care imply from an ethical perspective? What does the picture signify in terms of fair resource allocation in the rural setting?

Rurality has many attractions—lack of interference from other people, an opportunity to be independent, the chance to be close to nature—but it imposes some obstacles to ensuring the health of rural residents. As the preceding summary suggests, socioeconomic indicators, particularly level of education and income, that are known to be determinants of health status are less favorable in rural communities. Rurality is also associated with poorer-quality health care. Health promotion, acute and chronic disease management, and disaster management are all reported to be less adequate. Not surprisingly then, health status is worse as indicated by higher morbidity and mortality in rural settings. Beyond these measures, which are static or cross-sectional comparisons between rural and urban communities, longitudinal measurement is likely to show even greater disparities, due to the adversity imposed by instability of rural communities. Population loss or stasis in rural areas—while urban areas grow—makes planning, delivery, and funding of rural services precarious. Finally, that rural communities, although isolated, are present in societies throughout the world is important in ethical considerations. While many of these communities have unique features, they share many ethically relevant characteristics.

Arguably, this picture of multifaceted disadvantages stems from the low density and wide dispersion of rural residents—the quintessential features of rural living. Dispersion imposes distance from services and limited access. Wide dispersion entails few individuals within a geographic area; hence there are few within the vicinity to patronize a business, attend a school, use a health care facility, pay taxes, and vote in political elections.

But it is interesting to consider what importance we should assign to such low numbers. A given rural community may be small, but the total number of rural communities can in combination yield a substantial fraction of a nation's population. From the perspective of distributive justice, does it matter how large a fraction of the total population they represent? Should the aggregate number matter?

If the numbers matter, is it the size of an individual rural community or the magnitude of the rural population of a nation as a whole that should determine the quantity of resources that are allocated to rural services? Rural communities are located in small pockets of any given state, region, or province. In practical terms this poses a political disadvantage in any negotiation for services.

Let us take as a starting point that the morally relevant focus of ethical analysis is on the individual.[3] As with any other group of individuals in disadvantageous circumstances, we consider what a society owes a person located in a rural setting. If rural location poses a disadvantage for any given individual, the obligation to meet that individual's needs should not be a function of the number of others in like circumstances. Yet the pertinent characteristic of rurality is the geography of a community, a population-based characteristic. This is the key tension in considering what is owed to rural residents. Much of health care requires large organizational structures that are resource-intense. On reflection then, it would seem that what we owe a given individual should not be a function of how many individuals are in like circumstances, but from a practical standpoint the way we fulfill the obligation might vary according to population density. Thus, all other things being equal, it is fairest to expend an equivalent amount per capita on all individuals regardless of community size, but a rural community of a dozen individuals might warrant a mobile clinic staffed by a nurse practitioner who is skilled in primary care, while a rural community of several hundred might warrant a practitioner who is permanently stationed in that community.

Shifting from consideration of the importance of *numbers* of rural residents, we must address the *degree* of disadvantage that rural residents experience. Returning to the earlier description, wide dispersion and low population density are associated to varying degrees with disadvantageous features that are part of rurality. Rural populations are less likely to have employment opportunities either because employers are no longer present or have never been present. Rural residents are thus likely to be unemployed or self-employed, have low incomes, and be without employment benefits. Thus, as we have already noted, they are more likely to be without health insurance. They are likely to have poor access to other services such as educational facilities. Residents who have remained in a previously prosperous community are likely to be those who are older or less able to leave communities that have become stagnant. They are thus disadvantaged from many perspectives.

One could argue for analytically handling the many disadvantages in a variety of ways. Perhaps we should scale the aggregate degree of disadvantage in any particular rural community to establish the degree of priority to assign it. How might the efforts to address various rural populations then look? A community with many disadvantages would be assigned a more substantial number of resources than a community with fewer disadvantages.

Alternatively, one could argue for teasing apart the various disadvantages and treating them as nonaggregable. Considering disadvantages separately makes it possible to characterize them and give each appropriate weight and response. If a given community faces poverty, handle it as we would other low-income populations. If a community has a high proportion of an ethnic minority that faces obstacles in the dominant culture of a society, this difficulty should be addressed as a separate matter in an appropriate manner. For the rare rural community that is composed of wealthy individuals, only concern about the disadvantages imposed by geographic distance would need to be taken into account.

An additional characteristic that we have noted about rural communities is their instability. In such communities, one might ask: What is the best way to respond to instability? Is it better to focus on the status quo or facilitate change? How much priority should rural communities assign to delivery of services to the few individuals who remain and how much should they emphasize vocational rehabilitation and relocation? As a matter of procedural justice, how should this priority-setting process take place and who should be participating in it? Should all these decisions be in the hands of a rural community's residents, or should leadership of the state or province where the community is located have a large voice in such decisions?

Another major dimension regarding allocation decisions in rural communities concerns the extent to which resources should be earmarked for health care versus other social determinants of health that lie outside the health care sector. With a limited budget, should a rural community prioritize efforts to build infrastructure that might attract new employers—such as roads and schools—to try to revitalize and increase its economic base? Given what we know about the impact of income on health, might not the latter be the best thing a community could do? In a similar vein, should a rural community and the surrounding state or province emphasize tax policies that keep taxes low to attract new business or maintain tax rates on the high side to fund services to the population?

Selection of an Ethical Framework

Having considered how to characterize aspects of rural communities for the purpose of thinking about allocation decisions for rural health and health care, we should examine various theories of distributive justice to consider their implications for distributing resources to target the health of rural populations. Several theories are at our disposal; among them are libertarian, utilitarian, egalitarian, prioritarian, and contractarian theories of justice. While it is beyond the scope of this chapter to delineate and examine the application of each of these approaches in great depth, I mention the rationale of these theories and then focus briefly on some consequences of their application.[4]

A libertarian approach to distributive justice would argue that individuals should be free and unconstrained to pursue the good as they each see it, so long as their pursuits do not harm others, limit others' liberty (without their consent), or preclude the ability to honor agreements freely entered into. Each individual deserves those resources garnered through personal labor. Government should not impose constraints and should not redistribute societal resources for the sake of disadvantaged individuals to the extent that this imposes on individual liberty. Were one to take a libertarian approach, rural communities would be encouraged to emphasize self-care and banding together voluntarily among themselves to the extent that they share an interest in promoting their health. They might pool their financial resources to attract providers and fund health care facilities. The consequences for individual rural communities, given their financial constraints, would likely be meager resources to address their health care needs. This analytic approach may be defensible and hold promise for promoting the self-sufficiency of rural communities, but it may hold less promise for garnering a share of the larger societal resources to improve the difficult circumstances of rural communities and guaranteeing adequate health of their populations. It holds little promise for rural communities in terms of promoting their interests on a par with other communities and little value in engaging the rest of a nation's population in the concerns of its rural citizens.

A utilitarian approach would aim to achieve the greatest good for the greatest number of individuals. This theoretical approach would lead to the selection of policy options that maximize the balance of benefits over harms. So long as the sum of goods is maximized, the distribution is not paramount. This approach is likely to be disadvantageous to rural residents. Given the small number of rural individuals and the significant costs of helping them, it is unlikely that rural programs will yield the greatest aggregate good.

An egalitarian approach considers all humans to be equal and would aim for their equal treatment. An egalitarian approach may well lead to a distribution of resources that is helpful to rural residents. Yet selecting an egalitarian approach leaves many questions to resolve. What would one aim to equalize? Given the differences in baseline health status, insurance status, available health care personnel, and proximity and character of clinical facilities, one must choose what to equalize.

A prioritarian perspective focuses most on addressing the concerns of the worst off. In some sense this approach is similar to an egalitarian approach, in that egalitarian theories tend to focus on bringing the least-advantaged individuals up to some baseline. A justification for a prioritarian view, as expressed by Lu Ann Aday (2001), is a commitment to vulnerable individuals and populations based on the belief that human communities are both the origins of vulnerability and the remedy for it. Vulnerable populations are defined as being at risk of poor physical, psychological, or social health through harm or neglect by others. In considering the application of a prioritarian approach, we should ask whether rural populations should be considered vulnerable populations that deserve priority. To the extent that rural populations have demonstrated poorer health, the designation seems applicable. Is there any downside to such a designation? Would rural individuals and communities, who are used to being self-sufficient and staunchly independent, object? They have developed strategies for surviving in isolation. The thought that they face disadvantages and might possibly warrant consideration on this basis may seem to them an unwelcome and disturbing suggestion. But if rural populations were to be considered like any vulnerable population that deserves priority, we might aim to equalize the health status of this population and plan to allocate greater funds per capita than the average risk population to achieve this goal.

Among the most prominent theories of justice of the twentieth century is the social contractarian theory developed by John Rawls to counter the problem posed by utilitarian theory—its inability to plausibly address questions of fair distribution. Rawls argued that this problem could best be addressed by arranging the distribution of societal goods according to the way a group of rational individuals would distribute them were they to be placed behind a veil of ignorance where they do not know their own fate (Rawls 1971). They would be uninformed about whether they are likely to be in an advantageous or disadvantageous position in society. In this ignorant state, they are likely to arrange goods so that the worst-off individuals are disadvantaged as little as possible. Norman Daniels developed his theory of just health care based on this social contractarian approach, arguing that health care is a special good that is needed by everyone to guarantee fair equality of opportunity in life (Daniels 1985). What might rational individuals behind the veil of ignorance decide about the appropriate level of resources for rural populations? One might guess that they would give rural residents a fair share of resources, not knowing whether they are likely to be rural residents.

The theoretical approaches mentioned so far offer grounds for the demands that some may make on others in the name of justice. In relation to the issue at hand here, they give normative reasons why society ought to provide resources for the good of rural populations. We should consider one other approach that assumes individuals have the capacity for enlightened self-interest. Such a capacity will lead them to recognize that what is best for themselves entails consideration of what is good for others, something akin to what David Hume has proposed.[5] Were we to take this perspective and argue for enlightened self-interest, we could engage in a discussion about why it would be in the interest of a nation as a whole to guarantee the health of its rural citizens. To the extent that it is in a nation's self-interest, it would seem self-evident that meeting the health needs of rural communities should be given priority on several counts. One reason might be that it is essential to have a healthy population in the agricultural sector of the economy. Another reason, based on migration trends, is that some fraction of rural individuals will move to cities and that it is prudent to keep them healthy to reduce the burden of disease in the growing urban population. Or one could reason that it would be problematic to have a weak link in the public health sector. Low rates of treatment of infectious disease in rural communities might create a reservoir of infection that poses a risk for other segments of the population. But what if other priorities concern a nation more? If a nation does not see it as a matter of self-interest to give attention to the health of its rural population, then we might rely on the other theoretical justifications that compel us to address the needs of rural populations on the basis of distributive justice.

This synopsis of theoretical approaches to distributive justice indicates the variety of answers one might arrive at in assigning resources for meeting the health needs of rural populations. Because there are various possible theory-driven answers without definitive resolution or consensus, some have argued that resource allocation decisions ought to rest on fair procedure. Norman Daniels and Jim Sabin have articulated an approach to procedural justice called "accountability for reasonableness." Decisions about resource allocation might be judged to be fair if: (1) they are publicly accessible; (2) the rationale for setting limits is reasonable—appealing to evidence, reasons, and principles that are accepted as relevant by fair-minded people; (3) there is a mechanism for appeals; and (4) there is some regulation of this process (Daniels and Sabin 2002).

Can we develop a coherent ethical approach to allocating resources for guaranteeing the health of rural health populations that builds from these various theories? I suggest that we should aim for equal health outcomes for all populations. Funds for rural populations would be allocated to accomplish this goal. The amount to be spent per capita might be explicitly and transparently determined by the public. I take a similar approach here to the one suggested by David Degrazia in his argument for a fair health care system for the United States. Following his approach, I argue that while people may differ significantly with respect to their endorsement of particular theories of justice, most of them are likely to agree on the appropriate goals of health care (Mappes and Degrazia 2006). Accordingly, I suggest that attempting to achieve the goal of equal health outcomes, within the constraints of feasibility, is such a goal.

The goal of equal health outcomes or status has appeal. Precisely because rural communities have such different features from urban communities and because providing identical services would be so impractical, aiming for equal health status and attempting to modify various factors to reach this aim may well make sense. Alternatively, one might argue for equal funding for rural health care. This approach, however, seems unlikely to be workable because the many barriers to healthy rural populations are likely to make the cost of promoting the health of this population more expensive than doing so in the urban population. We might sacrifice some efficiency overall to provide rural communities with adequate core services and a greater chance of achieving health outcomes comparable with those in urban communities.

This reasoning relies largely on an egalitarian foundation. It incorporates a prioritarian perspective in that it assumes that to the extent that rural populations are more vulnerable, more should be spent on their behalf. It incorporates an element of procedural justice in that any excess expenditure per capita would be subject to public deliberation. There is some sacrifice of the utilitarian emphasis on maximal aggregate good, but the approach does not totally ignore emphasis on outcomes.[6]

Implications for Policy

The connection between ethically sound priorities and policy making is always tenuous. While many policy options are suggested here, it should be pointed out that in practice policy options actually get adopted only when a convenient, well-suited window of opportunity arises (Kingdon 2002). Furthermore, health policy reform cannot take place without attention to the political realm (Roberts et al. 2004). An examination of rural health policy in the United States suggests that it is motivated by a set of relative needs comprising shortages of health care professionals, lower payment for health services, and slower uptake of medical innovations (Ricketts 1999). These relative shortages are politically meaningful enough to drive the creation of programs to address them. This process reflects a lack of comprehensive health policy for rural health—let alone national health care—in general in the United States. Furthermore, without a comprehensive and equitable health care system, the creation of policies to address the needs of underserved populations is subject to the efforts of representatives who advocate for factions (Ricketts 1999). In this context, various constituents of the rural health system—be it hospitals, physicians, nurse practitioners, or others—argue for programs that support their funding and organizational structures. Above and beyond this mélange of interests, a voice for rural health interests has evolved in the United States based on convergent interests as exemplified by the National Rural Health Association. In the midst of such a chaotic picture, efforts to plan for rural health care have been catalyzed by the Office of Rural Health Planning (ORHP) in the Health Resources and Services Administration of the U.S. Department of Health and Human Services. The analysis of rural health care in the United States, published through the support of ORHP, is structured to match the perceived relative shortages in components of rural health care compared to metropolitan regions. Based on that analysis, policies are recommended to ameliorate the shortcomings of rural health care in the United States.

In countries with more centralized health systems, the planning of policies for rural health care is more straightforwardly organized. In Canada, efforts at coordinated planning for rural health services are carried out through the Office of Rural Health that was established by the Public Health Agency of Canada in 1998.[7] In the United Kingdom, experts have argued that an allowance should be made for sparsity in the allocation of resources to rural populations. Abhaya Asthana and colleagues suggest that there should be an adjustment for rurality by the National Health Service of England that should be made on several grounds: (1) the existing allocation formula introduces systematic bias in favor of urban areas in the way it expresses need for health care; (2) the system's method of compensating for unavoidable variations in costs of services takes insufficient account of the additional costs associated with rural services; (3) with an increasing emphasis on meeting national quality standards, rural services cannot practice lower levels of service; and (4) other U.K. countries have set a precedent of adjusting for rurality (Asthana et al. 2003).

In less developed countries or resource-poor countries, attention to the needs of rural populations is likely to address analogous concerns about the distribution of resources but reflect baseline conditions that are far more constrained. As developing countries struggle to achieve economic growth, rural communities are likely to fall behind unless particular attention is paid to the widening gap (Kahn and Yardley 2004). In recognition of this reality, the World Bank, at the invitation of the Chinese government, has studied rural health in China.[8] The Institute for Rural Health Studies in India recognizes the importance of a wide range of issues from the socioeconomic determinants of intrafamily food distribution to transportation to health facilities.[9]

The variety and complexity of health systems across many countries and the intricacies of policy making render it difficult to briefly consider the translation of the ethical analysis into policy. Suffice it to say that policy making requires sensitivity to political necessities of advocacy and attention to interest groups. Nonetheless, at the risk of offering suggestions that pay less than full attention to political realities, I consider what the preceding ethical analysis might imply regarding sound policy for resource allocation for rural health and health care.

Rural health policy should focus on the individual rural resident as the ethically relevant determinant of the amount of resources devoted to a rural community. A given rural individual deserves what he or she does regardless of the size of his or her community or the percentage of the national population that is rural.

The goal should be to achieve equal *health status* or health outcomes among rural and urban populations rather than planning to equalize *services* or *access*. We might aim for equal health outcomes within publicly determined and transparent financial limits regarding per capita expenditures. In other words, we might be willing to sacrifice some efficiency overall to provide rural communities with adequate core services and a greater chance of achieving comparable health outcomes with urban communities. In certain instances where rural populations have superior outcomes, we might seek a balance by spending comparably less. While political expediency may argue for the same number of health care providers or services per capita in rural and urban areas, there are several reasons why this may not be the best approach. While advocacy for equal services is a straightforward approach, the distinctive barriers in rural communities, such as the geographic and personnel limitations, and the potentially unique solutions, such as technological and organizational innovations, make it wise to plan unique strategies rather than following the urban mold. For example, a rural community may be better served by fewer physicians but with the addition of geospatial information technology. A rural community is better served not by aiming to have the same number of hospital beds per capita as a metropolitan area but rather by adding a mobile clinic and proficiently staffed emergency transport system. Policy should be attentive to the reality that the size of a rural community is relevant for selecting the types of services that might be best.

In allocating funds to programs, the priority assigned to programs should take into account the advantages of existing and cutting-edge technology and the best in evidence-based medicine to most efficiently achieve the goal of promoting rural health status. To that end, we should make services as mobile as possible by providing circulating services to rural populations.

Along with setting funding priorities, those who plan for the health of rural communities would be well advised to extend the value of personnel resources by creating regulatory and organizational environments that are conducive to the most effective rural care. Thus, we may need to loosen restrictions on the level of supervision required in order to extend care to populations in need. This has been done for dental hygienists (Krause, Mosca, and Livingston 2003), and it has been argued that it needs to be done for advanced practice nurses (Smyth 2003). Given the degree of interdependence among rural providers, we should aim to improve the working relationship among providers (Farmer, Stimpson, and Tucker 2003).

Looking beyond the health care sector, allocation of resources in rural communities should be balanced to promote the economic viability of the community along with efforts to design optimal health services. Thus, funding of rural communities aimed at maximizing the health status of its population should focus not only on the health sector but rather on a combination of health and other services, including education, vocational rehabilitation, and business improvement facilities. By allocating resources in this way, a rural community will balance the need to educate its population, attract business, offer job training and vocational rehabilitation, and address other factors that affect socioeconomic determinants of health with the delivery of efficiently designed health services.

Finally, rural health care leaders would do well to balance their focus on their own communities with a countervailing broader vision. Attention to strategies developed by rural communities around the world, adoption of techniques that have worked in other communities, and coordination of efforts with other communities may serve to make rural health care planning as farsighted and efficient as possible.

Conclusion

The circumstances of rural communities leave them susceptible to having fewer of the resources necessary to ensure health status on par with more heavily populated communities. In this sense, rural residents are more vulnerable and deserve priority in funding. Allocation of resources for rural communities would not necessarily be best guided by aiming for parity of services with urban communities because their unique geography precludes the possibility that similar services will yield similar results. Rather, allocation of resources for rural communities would be best guided by aiming for parity of health status and by taking advantage of innovations in communication and technology to achieve this goal.

NOTES

The views expressed here are those of the author and do not reflect the policies of the National Institutes of Health or the U.S. Department of Health and Human Services.

I would like to thank several readers from the Department of Clinical Bioethics, including Reidar Lie, Steve Pearson, David DeGrazia, and Emili Evans; commentators from the workshop on Rural Health Care, sponsored by the University of Nevada, Reno, particularly Craig Klugman; Patrick Gerland at the United Nations Population Division; and anonymous reviewers for their constructive criticism and suggestions.

1. The most recent online data (http://esa.un.org/wup/source/country.aspx [accessed February 25, 2008]) regarding rural and urban demographics released by the United Nations include the following short description:

> The definitions presented are generally those used by national statistical offices in carrying out the latest available census. When the definition used in the latest census was not the same as in previous censuses, the data were adjusted whenever possible so as to maintain consistency. In cases where adjustments were made in such a way as to ensure consistency with the definition used in previous censuses, that information is included in the sources . . . United Nations estimates and projections are based, to the extent possible, on actual enumerations. In some cases, however, it was desirable to incorporate official or other estimates of urban population size. When that is done, the sources of data indicate it. (United Nations Department of Economic and Social Affairs Population Division 2004, p. 111)

A version of the definition and methodology used can be found in *World Urbanization Prospects: The 2003 Revision,* pp. 103–4, available at www.un.org/esa/population/publications/wup2003/2003wup.htm (accessed February 25, 2008).

2. I quote here from the USDA Economic Research Service:

> According to official U.S. Census Bureau definitions, rural areas comprise open country and settlements with fewer than 2,500 residents. Urban areas

comprise larger places and densely settled areas around them. Urban areas do not necessarily follow municipal boundaries. They are essentially densely settled territory as it might appear from the air. Most counties, whether metropolitan or non-metropolitan, contain a combination of urban and rural populations.

Urban areas are of two types—urbanized areas and urban clusters—identical in the criteria used to delineate them but different in size. The Census Bureau defines an urbanized area wherever it finds an urban nucleus of 50,000 or more people. They may or may not contain any individual cities of 50,000 or more (152 currently do not). In general, they must have a core with a population density of 1,000 persons per square mile and may contain adjoining territory with at least 500 persons per square mile. Urbanized areas have been delineated using the same basic threshold (50,000 population) for each decennial census since 1950, but procedures for delineating the urban fringe are more liberal today. In 2000, 68 percent of Americans lived in 452 urbanized areas.

The same computerized procedures and population density criteria are used to identify urban clusters of at least 2,500 but fewer than 50,000 persons. This delineation of built-up territory around small towns and cities is new for the 2000 census. In 2000, 11 percent of the U.S. population lived in 3,158 urban clusters.

According to this system, rural areas consist of all territory located outside of urbanized areas and urban clusters. (USDA Economic Research Service 2007)

Canada and other countries in the Organization of Economic Cooperation and Development use definitions that are published by the Public Health Agency of Canada. See www.phac-aspc.gc.ca/rh-sr/paper_e.html.

3. In focusing on the individual as the unit of analysis, I do not mean to imply that the well-being of the individual should take precedence over the well-being of groups or communities. I do wish to give some weight to the claim that we should respect each and every individual regardless of circumstances. From an analytical standpoint, focusing on the individual is straightforward. If we were to compare what we owe rural and urban communities, then the differences in these types of communities and the relevance of these differences for allocation decisions is difficult to sort out.

4. Allen Buchanan (1989) provides a useful review of various theories of justice.

5. Larry Churchill suggests that we ought to take heed of David Hume's view of justice as an expression of self-interest. "The remedy for 'unequal affection,' or partiality, as Hume saw it, is not the counterbalancing of self-interest by another sentiment, like benevolence, but adherence to learned responses based on an assessment of where our true interests lie" (1994, p. 48).

6. Note that the analytic approach to resource allocation that I have just outlined with regard to the health of rural populations is not unique—one would apply a similar analysis to other pressing needs and vulnerable populations. It serves to logically consider the extent of overall expenditure that one might assign toward rural health. I should also note that this analysis does not address how assigned funds might be spent. Nor does it include many aspects of planning and coordination that are crucial to planning the delivery of services to populations. Some of these planning issues are considered in the next section on policy.

7. As the Canadian Office of Rural Health Web site states, "The Office provides policy advice on rural health issues; identifies rural health issues in relation to broad federal, departmental and regional priorities; fosters understanding about rural health issues of national concern and builds consensus on how to address them; identifies emerging trends; works with others to promote, encourage or influence action on rural health issues; and promotes the involvement of rural citizens, communities and health care providers" (Public Health Agency of Canada 2007).

8. See "Meeting China's rural health challenge," www.worldbank.org/china ruralhealth (accessed December 30, 2006).

9. See the Institute for Rural Health Studies Web site: www.irhs.org/Past_ research_projects.htm (accessed December 30, 2006).

REFERENCES

Aday, L. A. 2001. *At risk in America: The health and health care needs of vulnerable populations in the United States.* 2d ed. San Francisco: Jossey-Bass.

Asthana, S., A. Gibson, G. Moon, and P. Brigham. 2003. Allocating resources for health and social care: The significance of rurality. *Health and Social Care in the Community* 11 (6): 486–93.

Australian Institute for Health and Welfare. 2006. Impact of rurality on health. www.ainw.gov.au/ruralhealth/overview.cfm (accessed November 19, 2006).

Averill, J. 2003. Keys to the puzzle: Recognizing strengths in a rural community. *Public Health Nursing* 20 (6): 449–55.

Bagchi, S. 2006. Telemedicine in rural India. *PLoS Med* 3 (3): e82.

Buchanan, A. 1989. Health care delivery and resource allocation. In *Medical ethics,* edited by R. M. Veatch. Boston: Jones and Bartlett Publishers.

Churchill, L. 1994. *Self-interest and universal healthcare: Why well-insured Americans should support coverage for everyone.* Cambridge, MA: Harvard University Press.

Daniels, N. 1985. *Just health care.* Cambridge, MA: Cambridge University Press.

Daniels, N., and J. Sabin. 2002. *Setting limits fairly—Can we learn to share medical resources?* New York: Oxford University Press.

Drugger, C. W. 2004. An exodus of African nurses puts infants and the ill in peril. *New York Times,* July 12.

Fallacaro, M. D., and T. Ruiz-Law. 2004. Distribution of U.S. anesthesia providers and services. *AANA Journal* 72 (1): 9–14.

Farmer, J., P. Stimpson, and J. Tucker. 2003. Relative professional roles in antenatal care: Results of a survey in Scottish rural general practice. *Journal of Interprofessional Care* 17 (4): 351–62.

Faruque, F. S., S. P. Lofton, T. M. Doddato, and C. Mangum. 2003. Utilizing Geographic Information Systems in community assessment and nursing research. *Journal of Community Health Nursing* 20 (3): 179–91.

Gibb, H. 2003. Rural community mental health nursing: A grounded theory account of sole practice. *International Journal of Mental Health Nursing* 12 (4): 243–50.

Grumbach, K., L. G. Hart, E. Mertz, J. Coffman, and L. Palazzo. 2003. Who is caring for the underserved? A comparison of primary care physicians and nonphysician clinicians in California and Washington. *Annals of Family Medicine* 1 (2): 97–104.

Helling, T. S. 2003. The challenges of trauma care in the rural setting. *Missouri Medicine* 100 (5): 510–14.

Hoa, N. P., A. E. Thorson, N. H. Long, and V. K. Diwan. 2003. Knowledge of tuberculosis and associated health-seeking behaviour among rural Vietnamese adults with a cough for at least three weeks. *Scandinavian Journal of Public Health (Supplement)* 62:59–65.

Humphreys, J. S., J. A. Jones, M. P. Jones, D. Mildenhall, P. R. Mara, B. Chater, D. R. Rosenthal, N. M. Maxfield, and M. A. Adena. 2003. The influence of geographical location on the complexity of rural general practice activities. *Medical Journal of Australia* 179 (8): 416–20.

Huttlinger, K., J. Schaller-Ayers, and T. Lawson. 2004. Health care in Appalachia: A population-based approach. *Public Health Nursing* 21 (2): 103–10.

Janes, R., and A. Dowell. 2004. New Zealand rural general practitioners 1999 survey—Part 3: Rural general practitioners speak out. *New Zealand Medical Journal* 117 (1191): U815.

Jennett, P. A., L. Affleck Hall, D. Hailey, A. Ohinmaa, C. Anderson, R. Thomas, B. Young, D. Lorenzetti, and R. E. Scott. 2003. The socio-economic impact of telehealth: A systematic review. *Journal of Telemedicine and Telecare* 9 (6): 311–20.

Joliffe, D. 2006. The cost of living and the geographic distribution of poverty. USDA ERS Report. U.S. Department of Agriculture. www.ers.usda.gov/publications/err26/err26_reportsummary.pdf (accessed November 18, 2006).

Kabir, Z. 2003. Demographic and socio-economic determinants of post-neonatal deaths in a special project area of rural northern India. *Indian Pediatrics* 40 (7): 653–59.

Kahn, J., and J. Yardley. 2004. Amid China's boom, no helping hand for young Qingming. *New York Times,* August 1.

Kingdon, J. W. 2002. The reality of policy making. In *Ethical dimensions of health policy,* edited by M. Danis, C. Clancy, and L. R. Churchill. New York: Oxford University Press.

Kirkhorn, S., R. T. Greenlee, and J. C. Reeser. 2003. The epidemiology of agriculture-related osteoarthritis and its impact on occupational disability. *World Medical Journal* 102 (7): 38–44.

Krause, D., N. Mosca, and M. Livingston. 2003. Maximizing the dental workforce: Implications for a rural state. *Journal of Dental Hygiene* 77 (4): 253–61.

Labiris, G., M. Fanariotis, C. Christoulakis, A. Petounis, G. Kitsos, M. Aspiotis, and K. Psillas. 2003. Tele-ophthalmology and conventional ophthalmology using a mobile medical unit in remote Greece. *Journal of Telemedicine and Telecare* 9 (5): 296–99.

Mappes, T. A., and D. Degrazia. 2006. *Biomedical ethics.* 6th ed. Boston: McGraw Hill.

Marmot, M., and R. G. Wilkinson. 1999. *Social determinants of health.* New York: Oxford University Press.

Moore, J., D. Zelen, I. Hafeez, A. K. Ganti, J. Beal, and A. Potti. 2003. Risk-awareness of cutaneous malignancies among rural populations. *Medical Oncology* 20 (4): 369–74.

National Rural Health Association. 2006. *What's different about rural health care?* www.nrharural.org/about/sub/different.html. Accessed December 18, 2006.

Ovrill, A., and B. Stilwell. 2004. Health professionals and migration. *Bulletin of the World Health Organization* 82:571. www.who.int/bulletin/volumes/82/8/editorial10804html/en/index.html (accessed December 18, 2006).

Parker, R. L., and G. I. Martin. 2004. Neonates in Gadchiroli: Field trial of home-based neonatal care in rural India (1993–2003). *Journal of Perinatology* Suppl 1:S1–112.

Public Health Agency of Canada. 2002. Canada's rural health strategy: A one year review. www.phac-aspc.gc.ca/rh-str/ (accessed November 28, 2006).

———. 2007. Office of rural health. www.phac_aspc.gc.ca/rh-sr/index.html (accessed February 20, 2008).

Rawls, J. 1971. *A theory of justice.* Cambridge, MA: Harvard University Press.

Ricketts, T. C., III. 1999. *Rural health in the United States.* New York: Oxford University Press.

Roberts, M. J., W. Hsiao, P. Berman, and M. R. Reich. 2004. *Getting health reform right: A guide to improving performance and equity.* New York: Oxford University Press.

Rowley, T. D. 2006. The rural uninsured: Highlights from recent research. U.S. Department of Health and Human Services Health Resources and Services Administration. http://ruralhealth.hrsa.gov/policy/UninsuredSummary.htm (accessed December 18, 2006).

Sharma, S. K., P. Pradhan, and D. M. Padhi. 2001. Socio-economic factors associated with malaria in a tribal area of Orissa, India. *Indian Journal of Public Health* 45 (3): 93–98.

Smith, A. C., J. Batch, E. Lang, and R. Wootton. 2003. The use of online health techniques to assist with the delivery of specialist paediatric diabetes services in Queensland. *Journal of Telemedicine and Telecare* 9 Suppl 2:S54–57.

Smith, S. M., and N. C. Campbell. 2004. Provision of oncology services in remote rural areas: A Scottish perspective. *European Journal of Cancer Care* 13 (2): 185–92.

Smyth, P. E. 2003. Advanced practice nurses leading the way: A rural perspective introduction. *SCI Nursing* 20 (4): 269–71.

United Nations Department of Economic and Social Affairs Population Division. 2004. *World urbanization prospects: The 2003 revision.* New York: United Nations Press.

United Nations Development Program. 2005. China human development report. www.undp.org.cn/downloads/nhdr2005/NHDR2005_complete.pdf (accessed December 11, 2006).

United Nations Population Division. 2005. Urban and rural areas. www.un.org/esa/population/publications/WUP2005/2005urban_rural.htm (accessed December 18, 2006).

———. 2007. World urbanization prospects: The 2007 revision population database. www.esa.un.org/unup/ (accessed July 11, 2008).

U.S. Department of Agriculture. 2003. Rural education at a glance. USDA Economic Research Service. www.ers.usda.gov/publications/rdrr98/rdrr98_lowres .pdf (accessed November 27, 2006).

———. 2007. Measuring rurality: What is rural? USDA economic research service. www.ers.usda.gov/Briefing/Rurality/What is Rural/ (accessed February 20, 2008).

U.S. Department of Housing and Urban Development. 2006. Economic development resources. www.hud.gov/offices/cpd/economicdevelopment/programs/ rhed/gateway/econdev.htm (accessed November 24, 2006).

Vail, J. 2002. The family health and rural improvement program in Tari. *Papua New Guinea Medical Journal* 45 (1–2): 147–62.

Vallerand, A. H., J. M. Fouladbakhsh, and T. Templin. 2004. Self-treatment of pain in a rural area. *Journal of Rural Health* 20 (2): 166–72.

Weiping, Deng, Wang Ping, Wang Xiaohong, Long Ling, Ye Shifang, Guan Xiaojing, Du Yan, et al. 2006. *China statistical yearbook 2006.* Translated by F. Nailin, Z. Weisheng, H. Shenglong, Y. Liqi, S. Shaoying, X. Hui and G. Dong. Beijing, China: National Bureau of Statistics of China. www.stats.gov.cn/english/ (accessed December 18, 2006).

Whitener, L. A. 2005. Policy options for a changing rural America. U.S. Department of Agriculture. www.ers.usda.gov/AmberWaves/April05/pdf/april05_feature_ policyoptions.pdf (accessed December 19, 2006).

WHO Commission on Social Determinants of Health. 2005. Towards a conceptual framework and analysis and action on the social determinants of health. World Health Organization. www.naccho.org/topics/justice/documents/

WHOCommissionTowardsConceptualFrame.pdf (accessed November 28, 2006).

Woersching, J. C., and A. E. Snyder. 2003. Earthquakes in El Salvador: A descriptive study of health concerns in a rural community and the clinical implications, part I. *Disaster Management Response* 1 (4): 105–9.

Young, T. L., and C. Ireson. 2003. Effectiveness of school-based telehealth care in urban and rural elementary schools. *Pediatrics* 112 (5): 1088–94.

PART II

PRACTITIONERS' VOICES

In this section we hear from two physicians and one psychologist who have practiced in various rural settings in the western United States. Elwood Schmidt entered practice as a general physician after graduating from medical school in 1957. His 50-year career spanned rural areas of Arizona, Nevada, New Mexico and Texas. Louis Borgenicht completed his residency in pediatrics in 1971 and spent his first two years of practice on a Native American reservation in Wyoming. Dan Goodkind is a psychologist in the small town of Vernal, Utah. His practice began shortly after finishing training in 1997 and continues today.

Each was asked to write a narrative of their experiences in response to the following questions:

1. How long have you been practicing? How long have you practiced in the rural setting?
2. Briefly describe what makes your location "rural."
3. How did you come to practice in this location?
4. How does your practice differ from that of urban colleagues?
5. What are the ethical challenges faced by rural practitioners?
6. How has the issue of maintaining confidentiality challenged you?
7. Have you ever thought that perhaps you should not treat a client based on a conflict of interest, and, if so, what were the circumstances and how was [the issue] resolved?
8. How do you manage clients when they cannot pay for services?
9. What resources are available to you for resolving ethical dilemmas?

10. If your practice closed, how would it affect your community?
11. If your community has inadequate resources, how many more practitioners would be needed to fully meet the needs?
12. How has your view about what is ethical changed since practicing in the rural setting?
13. What do you think you have missed or gained by practicing in the rural setting?
14. What part of your academic training prepared you to practice in the rural setting?
15. How would you change the academic training to prepare for the rural setting? What other experience would have been useful?
16. What compels you to stay in the rural setting?

These three health care providers wrote about practicing in small rural towns and about the ethical issues they confronted such as culture shock, lack of resources, patients' access to care, value differences, and community responsibilities. Their narratives provide personal, firsthand accounts of life in rural practice, especially for those who may never have had such an experience.

CHAPTER 5

Reflections on Fifty Years in Rural Health Care

ELWOOD L. SCHMIDT, M.D.

Elwood L. Schmidt, M.D., began his career in 1957 as a general practitioner (GP) working for the U.S. Public Health Service, Division of Indian Health Services, in a small town in rural Arizona. In 1972, he became board certified in family practice. Dr. Schmidt practiced in rural areas of Arizona, Nevada, Texas, and New Mexico. Throughout most of his 50 years of practice, he often was the only physician or the only general practice physician in the area. He is now semiretired, working part-time in Lovelock, Nevada.

Training

I graduated from the University of Texas Medical Branch, Galveston, Texas, in June 1956 and then did a rotating internship at White Cross Hospital, Columbus, Ohio, through June 1957. On July 1, 1957, I began practice on duty with the U.S. Public Health Service, Division of Indian Health Services, in Keams Canyon, the headquarters for all services to the Hopi Indians of northern Arizona. Keams Canyon is located about 80 miles north of Holbrook and Winslow, Arizona. In 1957 the roads connecting all three towns were still dirt. I was one of two physicians there, although patient volume would have justified four physicians. After a year, I was assigned to duty in Schurz, Nevada, which is 100 miles southeast of Reno and 35 miles north of the nearest town of Hawthorne, Nevada. Schurz was a two-physician station with an outpatient clinic and inpatient hospital beds, serving the medical needs of the Paiute, Shoshone, and Washoe tribes of Western Nevada, as well as Indians in Yerington, Fallon, Lovelock, Moapa, and Reno, and boarding school residents at Stewart Indian School in Carson City, Nevada. The service population spanned more than 150 miles in several directions, so access was not always convenient for our patients.

I decided to practice in small towns because I realized that choice of a practice location is not as simple as it may first seem; economics plays a big part. I started with romantic notions about small-town life and stayed because being the big frog in a small pond is seductive. In July 1959, I went into private practice in Slaton, Texas, about 18 miles southeast of Lubbock, Texas, where I remained for two years until 1961. Slaton was a town of 6,000 with a Catholic hospital in place. That it was rural was locally defined, at least in part, by the amount of time it took for a trip to Lubbock, as well as the attitude of the largely farming population. If a physician referred a patient to a specialist in Lubbock, he always ran the risk of being thought lacking in essential capabilities, as most people wanted and expected the GP to know everything and to be able to perform all except the most complicated surgeries. As a young physician, I knew nothing of the business of medicine. Office visits were two or, occasionally, three dollars. I joined an established practice and was able to learn the bare rudiments of medical business practices from the one physician and his office staff. The town was a reasonably prosperous farming and railroad community, so there was a chance most people would be able to pay me for services and treatment.

The same attitude and expectations were held by the 4,000 people in Jal, New Mexico, where I practiced from 1961 to 1972. For 8 of those 11 years, I was the only doctor in town with a hospital of 14 beds to be manned 24/7/365. The nearest towns were Eunice, New Mexico, 25 miles north with a population of 4,000 and Kermit, Texas, 25 miles south with a population of 8,000. In comparison to Jal and Eunice, Kermit was rich in medical resources, as it had a general surgeon, an orthopedist, and a pediatrician. Jal was a company town where most of the people were employed by El Paso Natural Gas Company and covered by the company health insurance, which was considered generous at the time. An office call was three dollars from 1961 to 1970 and then went to four dollars. For an appendectomy I was paid $150, a tonsillectomy $75, and deliveries $130, which included all prenatal care, postnatal care, and newborn care, plus the routine labs. This amount was considered a good rate of pay in those days.

After 11 years, I left Jal in March 1972, and continued my practice in Yuma, Arizona, a town of 42,000 people. Yuma was primarily agricultural industries and retired folks from "up north." Yuma was considered rural by geography. It was 180 miles east to the comparatively larger town of Phoenix, Arizona, and 180 miles west and over the mountains to San Diego, California. The Yuma practice was also rural as defined by the poor physician-to-population ratio. There were 11 GPs, four general surgeons, three radiologists, two urologists, and one internist.

Rural/Urban Differences

Though there are big differences between small- and big-town medical practices, I'm not sure the differences are as large today as they were 30 to 50 years ago. In a rural community the physician is known by everyone. The physician is identified and individually held responsible for the treatment and results. In a larger town, a physician in a solo or group practice can easily remain anonymous. Repeatedly, I have seen that patients in a larger town have only the vaguest idea of who they consulted: "It was one of the doctors at the XYZ Clinic. I don't remember the name." In a small rural town, they always knew that it was Dr. Schmidt who treated them. This lack of anonymity seems to frighten many doctors away from rural practice. In addition, consulting with specialists and colleagues is more difficult in the rural setting. In a large group setting, one learns informally from casual conversations with peers. Such absorption of knowledge is unobtainable in a small rural practice.

Ethical Issues

There is definitely more awareness of ethical issues in 2007 versus in 1957, 1967, 1977, or even 1987. Part of this increased awareness is because of medical advances that make end-of-life issues pertinent. The hospice movement has helped to articulate approaches to death that did not really intrude on many of us previously, particularly in rural practice. In 1957, and for many years thereafter, the view was "I'm the doctor and I know what is good for you and you should do what I tell you to do." In my experience, the issues of autonomy and other aspects of ethical practice began to invade our consciousness only in the late 1970s, when the hospice movement was first gaining ground and resuscitation and life-prolonging therapies were becoming more available and more widely used.

Physician Impairment

One of the biggest ethical problems I saw was the matter of the impaired physician. Alcoholism was rife in our West Texas / southeastern New Mexico medical community and was winked at, ignored, and even accepted by us and our patients. Nowadays, we would consider not reporting the impaired doctor to the medical licensing authority unethical and probably illegal. The impaired physician was protected by the fact that if we didn't have a bad doctor to cover for us, we had no doctor.

Lower Standards of Practice

The single greatest and most repeated ethical error I have seen in the four Western states in which I practiced over the past 50 years has been the belief that rural medical practice should be held to a lower standard than that of a bigger city. This view prevailed among many physicians, patients, and rural city fathers—the mayors and members of the chambers of commerce who were enthusiastic in their pursuit of doctors for their towns. The city fathers frequently had some political clout countywide and statewide and would lobby vigorously for licensure for a doctor willing to come to their town. Any objections raised by other physicians were quickly dismissed: "You just want to keep all the patients for yourselves" was the fathers' view. The local residents' view was that small-town care does not have to meet prevailing standards. I have too often seen physicians trained in a specialty set off to practice in a small town with the attitude that their training in cardiology, or whatever else, has prepared them to deal with the multitude of human ailments that they have not considered, whether it is orthopedic, pulmonary, psychiatric, pediatric, dermatological, or whatever. Prepared general (family) practice physicians should have at least exposed themselves to these fields, be able to recognize the resources available to them, and know their limitations within those fields. The rural physician must always resist the idea that because he or she is in a small town he or she can practice *small-town,* otherwise known as inferior, medicine.

For example, in 1969 a new doctor came to Eunice, New Mexico, from Jal 25 miles away. I was briefly delighted with the thought that once again I might be able to trade off coverage and have a free weekend. The idea of entrusting the care of my patients to him evaporated quickly when I learned that he had been dismissed from four different orthopedic residencies, none of which would have prepared him for a general medical practice in a rural setting. He had been let go from one program for unspecified acts of cruelty. The head of another of the residency programs told me in a phone conversation that the doctor had deficiencies, but he could probably handle "taking care of colds and stuff like that in general practice." I thought that comment showed overwhelming ignorance on the part of an Ivy League teaching institution regarding what a doctor in a small New Mexico town would face on a daily basis. Later, a medical board investigation of the new doctor ensued after multiple inappropriate surgeries—15 knee operations on teenaged girls in a population of 3,000, a disproportional number. Also, the number of appendectomies he performed on local young women that had normal tissue findings was out of line with practice standards.

Access to Health Care

In my experience, access to health care was always an issue for patients and physicians in small towns. Interpersonal differences had to be put aside in consideration of the fact that as the only doctor in town you had to provide care to everyone. I also felt an obligation to provide service regardless of patients' ability to pay. I knew the circumstances of most of the people I saw and did not truly mind serving those unable to pay. My benevolence was challenged, however, by those who cashed their medical insurance check and used the proceeds to fund a trip to Las Vegas or bought an extra shotgun but didn't bother to pay me. After 11 years in practice in Jal, New Mexico, I was owed more than $45,000 in three- and four-dollar visit fees. A simple thank-you and acknowledgment of appreciation for my care might be all the recompense I would receive.

Confidentiality

Confidentiality is always a problem in a small town because one's friends and neighbors work in the hospital or doctor's office. However, my experience has been that the government is much more concerned about their version of confidentiality than 97 percent of my patients. I believe that HIPAA regulations have severely restricted the sharing of essential medical information among doctors. When a doctor in the ER in Lovelock, Nevada, is faced with a patient recently discharged from one of the hospitals in Reno and cannot learn any of the lab values, x-ray results, or other essential information because of HIPAA regulations, the value of confidentiality is nil. This sort of withholding of information is dangerous.

The Loss of Great Certitude

Ethical dilemmas in rural practice, or any practice, must first be recognized as dilemmas before they can be addressed by reflection or consultation. I'm not sure that in the day-to-day setting of clinical practice, now or 45 years ago, that I or my physician colleagues recognized ethical dilemmas as such. In the 1950s and 1960s and even later in West Texas and southeastern New Mexico, a moral or ethical question would most likely be addressed by a fundamentalist Christian pastor and answered from within that ethos. And there would be great certitude in the answer. Today, there may be more recognition of ethical issues, but there is also less certainty about what to do about them.

CHAPTER 6

Serving the Underserved

Personal, Social, and Medical Challenges

LOUIS BORGENICHT, M.D.

Louis Borgenicht, M.D., began his career as a pediatrician working for the Indian Health Service (IHS) of the U.S. Public Health Service (USPHS) on the Wind River Reservation in Arapahoe, Wyoming. He faced the dual challenges of learning to be a new primary physician with few of the resources afforded urban medical teaching facilities while also living and working in a culturally unfamiliar environment.

Part of my decision to practice in a rural environment was related to the fact that I was training in medicine during the Vietnam War. I had a near miss going to war when my 1A classification—must report for military service in Vietnam—came during the final week of my first year of medical school. My wife hid the draft card from me until I completed my exams. I was convinced it had been a political reclassification because along with a long list of medical students and physicians, I had signed an antiwar petition that appeared prominently in the *New York Times*.

Toward the end of my San Francisco pediatric internship in June 1970, I realized that I would not have to confront the Vietnam War personally. My salvation was being accepted as a general medical officer in the U.S. Public Health Service (USPHS). I would be stationed for two years on the Wind River Indian Reservation in Arapahoe, Wyoming. Having grown up as a nice Jewish boy from the suburbs of New York and having been lucky enough to experience the post-1960s hip culture of San Francisco during my internship, I realized my family and I were in for two years of culture shock. We would be neither members of the Wyoming cowboy culture in Riverton, where we rented a house, nor members of the Arapahoe society on the reservation.

I also faced a significant personal challenge with the local medical culture. I would be sharing night call with the Riverton Memorial Hospital general practitioners, many of whom did not like taking care of Native American patients. Some of the local physicians were unabashedly racist. As believers in small government and the free market, local doctors saw me as a representative of government medicine. My presence seemed a threat to the sanctity of their private practices.

Challenges for the New IHS Physician

Even before I began my commission with USPHS, I began to think about clinical and ethical issues I had not yet confronted in my training. First, there was the issue of responsibility. Although medical internship is geared to enable trainees to gradually assume greater degrees of confidence and responsibility, my experience in the Indian Health Service (IHS) would be the first time I would be on my own making decisions about patients' health. I would likely be there for only two years and, like other officers before me, might be seen as a short-timer, putting my need to avoid service in Vietnam over and above the health care needs of the reservation. Some Arapahoes were fiercely patriotic: Would they see me as a privileged draft dodger?

Then there were the cultural issues to discover. How did the beliefs of this particular group of Native American tribes affect their interaction with allopathic medicine? Did they think of illness as a short-term problem that could be fixed with medication? Or did they see illness as a chronic condition which must be endured and cannot be cured? Or was their view of illness based on traditional Arapahoe beliefs and corresponding remedies?

Finally, there were issues to consider resulting from the fact that the IHS was a federal bureaucracy. Would there be constraints on the services I could provide my patients as a result of funding cuts or program curtailments? I was frustrated in my efforts to discover relevant issues confronted by previous physicians. Literature on the IHS was sparse if not nonexistent. A year after I left the IHS, Robert and Rosalie Kane (1972) published *Federal Health Care (With Reservations).* The Kanes had been stationed at

Shiprock, New Mexico, a setting much different from Wyoming, but their experience with government bureaucracies was similar. I sated my cultural curiosity by reading literature on contemporary Native American activism. My favorites were the bestselling *Bury My Heart at Wounded Knee* by Dee Brown (1971) and *Akwesasne Notes,* a politically active Native American newspaper.

Finding My Own Style

There were five medical officers on the reservation, and each adopted an approach to caring for the Arapahoes. One physician made it clear from the beginning that he intended to cater to the Native Americans because as a white man sympathetic to them, he was interested in being assimilated into their culture. While seeing myself as someone with a cultural consciousness, I simply wanted to practice medicine and earn my patients' respect. My approach led to the Arapahoe accepting and respecting me as a medical doctor. One of the community health aides (CHAs) spoke to me over lunch about the fact that I was not giving antibiotics to patients with colds. She indicated that some of the patients were miffed, feeling that I was denying them something they deserved and needed. I told the CHA what I told all my patients—that antibiotics were unnecessary for most upper respiratory infections and might even be harmful. The interesting thing was that after several months my relationship with most of my patients changed; they seemed to accept my medical judgment.

My presence in Riverton, Wyoming, as a general medical officer in the IHS posed a unique dilemma. Until I was stationed at the Arapahoe Clinic in July 1971, the only health care available to most Native Americans on the Wind River Reservation was 34 miles away on the western end of the reservation at Fort Washakie or in the emergency rooms of two small community hospitals in Riverton (eight miles away) or Lander (18 miles away). The doctors at Riverton Memorial Hospital were by and large politically conservative, and several of them were members of the John Birch Society. Their antipathy toward the Native Americans was both political—the Native Americans were served by a free health care system that the doctors saw as government medicine—and racial—Riverton was a cowboy town with a distinctly western ethic and the Native Americans were viewed as poor and drunk. There were certain ironies about living in a cowboy town and taking care of Native Americans. Alcohol and its attendant violence was a staple of life in Riverton, and each incident seemed to reinforce the stereotypes by which Indians were viewed by the Anglo community. Riverton had a definite redneck flavor, both politically and from the perspective of lifestyle—gun racks in the back of the pick-ups, western wear, and a swagger to the stride of those who felt the West belonged to them and not the Native Americans. Early on I made the egregious error of walking into a bar on Main Street in a blue suit and tie. My wife and I had been out to dinner at a steak restaurant with some friends. Luckily, one of my neighbors recognized me and ushered me to a back corner. My garb was definitely inappropriate, and I never wore it again. As one who served and advocated for the Native Americans, I was already suspect.

As a member of the medical staff in Riverton, my position was at times difficult. One morning I made rounds at the hospital and discovered an 18-month-old child admitted for dehydration who was receiving clysis. I had never heard of this approach to hydration and was shocked to discover it was provided by placing a needle subcutaneously to administer fluids. The usual method was intravenous. When I broached the subject with the physician involved he got defensive and angry. "What did you expect me to do?" he yelled. "I couldn't find a suitable vein. Besides, I had other patients to take care of. IHS should have called you. Those Indians are your patients!" The frustration and antipathy this particular doctor demonstrated were not uncommon among the medical staff there and added some degree of difficulty to my two years in the IHS. The major medical problems I encountered there were attitudinal, and I could not broach many subjects with the medical staff. They viewed me as a bleeding-heart liberal rather than the ombudsman I perceived myself to be.

Frontier Medicine

Having come from an urban, academic medical environment, I occasionally found the rural setting daunting. Although I did have colleagues on the reservation and one other pediatrician to consult about medical dilemmas, the resources of an urban medical center were simply not available. One afternoon a four-year-old Native American boy came into my clinic with fever, tachycardia, and shortness of breath. He was acutely ill and clearly in some degree of distress. He had a loud holosystolic murmur and signs of congestive failure. A week earlier he had been treated for strep throat. I realized he had acute rheumatic fever—the first case I had ever seen—and arranged for his admission to the local hospital until he could be transferred to the government hospital in Denver. I spent the night at the Riverton hospital watching him and stabilizing him with the help of the doctors in Denver via the telephone. It felt like frontline or at least frontier medicine and was both frightening and rewarding. This experience was made even more intense by the fact that I was the responsible physician. Ultimately, the boy recovered, and I learned how to work in the context of limited resources.

Despite these challenges, had I not been married I would likely have stayed beyond my two-year obligation to the USPHS. The experience of those two years was hard on my wife with two young boys aged one and three, occasional winters of 40 degrees below zero, and a cultural environment unlike any she had experienced. Years later she admitted to me that she thought she had leukemia at the time. Most likely, she was depressed.

Many years have passed since my experience on the reservation. Looking back now, I can say that it was exciting, novel, and rewarding on personal, medical, and social levels. This experience may have led me to be interested in medical service to the underserved. In 1996, I spent two weeks in Nepal with Interplast—a humanitarian organization that provides reconstructive surgery for children. I hope to repeat that experience when I retire.

REFERENCES

Brown, D. 1971. *Bury my heart at Wounded Knee: An Indian history of the American West.* New York: Holt, Rinehart and Winston.

Lane, R. L., and R. A. Kane. 1972. *Federal health care (with reservations).* New York: Springer.

CHAPTER 7

Ethical and Sociocultural Issues in Rural Mental Health Care

DAN GOODKIND, PH.D.

Dan Goodkind, Ph.D., is a clinical psychologist who has practiced for 10 years in Vernal, Utah. After completing his doctorate in 1997, Dr. Goodkind practiced briefly in rural eastern Tennessee before moving to northeastern Utah. He is the owner and director of the Ashley Family Clinic. Dr. Goodkind discusses his experiences practicing clinical psychology in rural settings, including his perspectives on ethical challenges in his professional and his personal life in a small town.

I began working professionally as a counselor with teenagers approximately twenty years ago in Santa Cruz, California. I then practiced in several rural settings in east Tennessee, including a rural mental health center in Hamblen County and the Brushy Mountain Prison in Morgan County. For a short time, I worked at a remote, mountainous, one-store town in Claiborne County, which borders on Tennessee, Kentucky, and Virginia. After working for about six months at a rehabilitation hospital in Kingsport, Tennessee, I moved to northeastern Utah. I have lived and practiced in Vernal since late 1997. My wife and I have settled here and now have two children. I worked at the regional public mental health center between 1997 and 2000, at which point I went into private practice.

Geographically, Vernal is a rural region because of the low population density and its distance from large metropolitan areas. The Uintah Basin, within which Vernal is located, is made up of three frontier counties: Daggett, Duchesne, and Uintah. This catchment area has a total land area of

8,413 square miles, with a population density of between eleven and twelve persons per square mile. The geography of the Uintah Basin is diverse and ranges between high mountainous and forested terrain to rich farmland and high desert. Vernal is located three hours east of Salt Lake City and two-and-a-half hours northwest of Grand Junction, Colorado. Historically, this region has been isolated. When I moved here, I was the first psychologist ever to have lived and practiced in the area.

Economically, I consider this area rural because so many residents make their living in one way or another off of the earth. Uintah County's economy rests on farming, ranching, and the removal of oil and gas. The local economy is increasingly influenced by worldwide energy prices. Currently, we are in the midst of an economic boom because of oil and natural gas exploration. The area feels less and less rural because of the increasing growth and material wealth here. Modern communication technologies, the growth of the mail order industry, and the Internet all contribute to this less-rural feeling. Of course, these technological and cultural changes are widespread. The most modest and run down of dwellings are as likely to have satellite dishes as to have old and rusting vehicles on the premises.

Family and community ties are important here, and rural individuals are more likely to deal with their problems through the family and church rather than seek professional or outside assistance. This area is blue collar. There is not a strong emphasis on education, and many young people never move away. Whatever differences may have existed between urban and rural areas are becoming smaller. Rural as well as urban teenagers play video games, have MySpace pages, and mimic the images and the attitudes depicted in the media.

Rural Practice

I was attracted to this particular area because of an available position through the National Health Service Corps (NHSC), the natural beauty of the region, and the region's obvious need for a child psychologist. The NHSC helped me and my wife repay our student loans. Although I might have taken a job here even without the student loan repayment, if not for the NHSC, I never would have discovered the job opportunity. I had done a rural practicum experience as part of my medical training, and this experience was what primarily prepared me for practice in the rural setting.

From the start, there has been more work here than I have been able to handle on my own. After entering into private practice in 2000, I opened a mental health clinic to add more mental health professionals. Vernal now has three psychologists (including myself), two clinical social workers, and an adult psychiatrist, whom we share with one of the local hospitals. A rural psychologist, like a rural family physician, is pressed to work with a wide variety of clinical conditions and patients of all ages. There is less of this pressure now that we have a clinic, but my clinical practice still has a lot of variety. I enjoy applying psychological diagnostic skills to different problems, and I work with children as well as with adults. I think it is still fair to state that, in general, rural people are somewhat less psychologically sophisticated and less comfortable discussing intimate personal matters than are urbanites. This discomfort can be both an obstacle and an opportunity for psychologists.

Clark D. Campbell and Michelle C. Gordon (2003) suggest that there may be characteristics common to rural psychologists. They are comfortable with a rural lifestyle, take active steps to integrate into the community, have broad general practices, are comfortable with a relatively high profile in the community, and have a higher tolerance for blurring of personal and professional boundaries. Although I have no hard data on this issue, these characteristics are certainly consistent with my observations of what is required to be successful in a rural practice setting.

Dual Roles

Perhaps the most obvious differences with regards to rural versus urban practice have to do not with the clinical work per se but with factors related to living in a small town. If you live in an urban neighborhood or suburb, it is less likely that you frequently run into patients during trips to the grocery store or to the gym. For a rural practitioner, these encounters are a daily occurrence. There is much less anonymity in rural areas.

This close social contact is a direct consequence of geographic isolation and limited economic resources. Thus, the most frequently identified ethical issue associated with rural psychology practice is having relationships with clients outside of role boundaries established by the psychotherapist-client relationship. Relationships in small towns cannot be neatly segmented and defined by social or professional roles because people see and interact with each other in a variety of settings. Therefore, the ethical pro-

hibition against dual relationships must be weighed against the consequences of refusing to provide treatment.

Living in the same small community with one's patients is a mixed
blessing. There is richness and satisfaction that comes from living among
individuals whom one has known in an intimate and meaningful way. I
find it especially satisfying when children with whom I have worked go
on to do well as teenagers and adults, and return to say hello, or smile
when they see me. However, the amount of private information that a rural
psychologist accumulates over time, concerning not only patients but also
their families, leads to uncomfortable situations in which one knows too
much about his neighbors. You simply have to keep your mouth shut. At
times, I feel somewhat distant and removed from other people in my community because of my role as a confidante and because I am reluctant to
let my guard down.

I will not work with someone if there is a close personal or professional
relationship or if there is too much proximity. This caveat was much more
problematic before Vernal had the clinic. There were situations when I
was pressured to work with someone when I would have preferred not to
because there were no good referral options. On one occasion, I was seeing
a man who was a professional acquaintance, and he lived directly across
the street from me. This situation became particularly awkward when he
reunited with his wife and they were having serious marital problems. To
make matters worse, he worked for another professional acquaintance,
who happened to be my next door neighbor, and there were issues between
them. I didn't want to go into my own front yard for quite a few months.
We ended up moving, which pretty much resolved the problem.

In addition, there have been numerous occasions when I have worked
with professional acquaintances as clients. We have always discussed potential problems beforehand. To my knowledge, dual relationships never
created a problem for my clients, but I have felt uncomfortable in meetings
and social gatherings when a patient or a family member of a patient has
been present.

Ethical Issues

I always knew ethical issues were important, but I did not know to
what degree until I started practicing. I've come to realize that ethical
sensitivity and personal integrity are vital in mental health practice. This

ethical attention is even more salient in a rural area. I've seen practitioners succeed and fail based largely on their ethics. When I was in graduate school, one of my professors stated that ethical issues are the most important determinants of our success or failure as clinical psychologists. I didn't understand him then, but I do now.

Payment

When clients cannot afford to pay for services, the problem is no different here than in urban areas. I work for a private clinic and do not receive government subsidies for operating expenses, so there are limitations in terms of how far I can lower fees. The clinic contracts with government entities that subsidize treatment for specific high-need populations, for example, children and youth in foster care and disabled adults who are receiving vocational rehabilitation services. We probably have more such government contracts than similar size group practices in urban areas because of the lack of services in this area relative to the needs in the community. Insurance reimbursement helps a lot of working-class patients to afford psychological treatment when otherwise they would not get help or would discontinue after only a few sessions.

Ethics Resources

The same resources regarding ethical dilemmas are available to me in Vernal as are available to any psychologist. I can refer to the ethical guidelines for our profession, do an online literature search on the problem, and/or consult with my colleagues. Professional consultation is critical when faced with an ethical dilemma. When living and practicing in a rural area, it is more difficult to develop relationships with other professionals, which makes participating in state and/or national professional organizations that much more critical. To me, there are no good excuses for not having resources when confronted with ethical dilemmas.

Standards of Care

Our clinic professionals maintain standards of care comparable to those at private clinics in urban areas. Ten years ago, the bar was set low with regard to mental health care in this community. Some individuals and families would make a six-hour round trip into Salt Lake City to receive professional mental health care, and others did not seek professional help because they could not make that trip and did not have good options available to them locally. The same individuals and many others now have local access to psychological and psychiatric care in the community. If our mental health clinic closed, certainly fewer of our residents would receive quality mental health services, and many would likely go without such services regardless of their needs (see chap. 2).

A Pretty Good Place

I've alluded to the main benefits and liabilities of rural practice. There is a large need for services in most rural communities. Our greatest need in the Uintah Basin is for a child psychiatrist. If a practitioner does a good job, he or she receives a lot of positive feedback, and it is easier to see the results of one's work in a small town. I feel that the drawbacks are primarily social for me and my wife, and educational for our children. I wish that there were more college-educated people and like-minded people (whom I have not treated) with whom I could have friendships.

The scenic beauty and lack of congestion as well as the benefits that I've previously mentioned are the compelling reasons I have stayed in a rural community. I have a five-minute commute to work. There is a lot to do outdoors, and overall it is a pretty good place to raise a family.

REFERENCE

Campbell, C. D., and M. C. Gordon. 2003. Acknowledging the inevitable: Understanding multiple relationships in rural practice. *Professional Psychology: Research and Practice* 34 (4): 430–34.

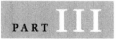

SPECIFIC ETHICAL ISSUES
AND SOLUTIONS

In this section of the book, the authors offer their perspectives and experiences dealing with specific ethical issues in rural practice and offering potential solutions to these concerns. Chapter 8, by Denise Niemira, looks at how standards developed for urban health care providers can be impossible to meet in the different cultural setting of rural practice where patients are often older, poorer, and sicker than in urban areas. Frank Chessa and Julien S. Murphy suggest in chapter 9 that a possible solution to ethical problems in low-density states might be the notion of a bioethics network where health care institutions share resources and expertise across a wide geographic area. In chapter 10, Elizabeth Thomas shows that sometimes the best intentions can have unforeseen negative consequences. Changes in welfare reform meant to bring more people into the work force have, in rural areas, had the effect in some cases of creating a social structure undercut by structural violence.

In chapter 11, Winslade and Beard-Duncan examine the challenges Texas faces in providing care to a scattered rural senior population. Anderson and Klugman suggest in chapter 12 that one way to improve rural medical care is to make rural practice more attractive to medical students and to provide support for rural practitioners by linking them more closely to the medical schools.

CHAPTER 8

Ethical Dimensions of the Quality of Rural Health Care

DENISE NIEMIRA, M.D.

In the new medical landscape, providing care is necessary but not sufficient. The new challenge is to provide high-quality health care to everyone who wants or needs it. The Institute of Medicine (IOM) has initiated a major campaign focused on systemic and systematic change to improve the quality of health care delivered to all Americans. In 2001, the IOM published *Crossing the Quality Chasm: A New Health System for the Twenty-First Century,* a report that offers a blueprint for restructuring the health care system to provide care that meets patient needs and is based on the best scientific evidence. The strategy calls for a commitment to six aims: "specifically, health care should be safe, effective, patient-centered, timely, efficient and equitable" (Institute of Medicine 2001, p. 6). The IOM proposes ten rules for redesigning and improving care to actualize these aims.

The publication of such specific rules by the prestigious IOM has ramifications for rural health care. This report provides a standard for approaching quality of care grounded in evidence-based decision making and raises ethical issues in clinical practice when the standard cannot be met or when application of the standard at the social and individual level creates conflict. This chapter explores how quality-of-care issues may present ethical dilemmas in rural practice.

This chapter is not intended as an exhaustive review of all possible dilemmas related to quality of care in rural practice. Nor is it intended to critically examine the rules proposed by the IOM or the use of evidence-based medicine as a basis for evaluating quality of care in general or in rural areas specifically. Others have undertaken the task of examining these issues (Gifford 1996; Grol 2001; Hofer et al. 1999; Stirrat 2004) and addressing specific agendas for quality improvement in rural health care (Calico et al. 2003; Rosenblatt 2002). The issue examined here is the need to evaluate the care practitioners deliver and how it meets the needs of the patient, physically and psychosocially. We can call this need quality of care, or we can call it part of the physician's obligation to the patient.

Quality as Part of Health Care

Before proceeding to case scenarios, I briefly explore two issues related to the concept of the quality of health care: Who or what are the determinants of the quality of health care, and what ethical principles or concepts are embodied in it?

Quality of health care, like quality of life, is an elusive concept that is highly value-laden (see chaps. 3 and 4). It is perhaps easiest to approach it operationally, defining the elements or properties that must be present and/or the processes that must be employed to be able to define the health care rendered as quality care. The IOM specifies the attributes of quality and offers a set of rules for guiding interested parties in getting there. These attributes (listed above) and rules (listed below in short form) specify a prevailing vision of quality and provide a locus in which to examine the questions raised:

1. Care based on continuous healing relationships
2. Customization based on patients' needs and values
3. The patient as the source of control
4. Shared knowledge and the free flow of information
5. Evidence-based decision making
6. Safety as a system property
7. The need for transparency
8. Anticipation of needs
9. Continuous decrease in waste
10. Cooperation among clinicians (Institute of Medicine 2001, pp. 8–9)

Implicit in these aims and rules is a notion of quality determined by at least two sets of data—objective knowledge that is evidence based and subjective appreciation that is consumer based. Thus quality is determined in relation to measurable standards by which one can say, "this care meets, fails to meet, or exceeds these standards," as well as in relation to personal perceptions by which one can say, "my care was good, poor, or excellent." In the ideal world, the objective and subjective determinants are aligned, and care that embodies best practices is perceived as such by its recipients. But the real world is not ideal, and consumers who pursue their own vision of health care outside the realm of standard medical practice may have needs and wants that are not evidence based. This creates the likelihood of tension and conflict between the two determinants and a less precise and consistent notion of quality, one that involves a balancing act or compromise when disagreement occurs. At the same time, these dual measures provide a richer notion of quality than sterile adherence to a set of practice guidelines. The IOM document acknowledges this tension in a telling statement: "The patient is always right, but sometimes the doctor knows better" (Institute of Medicine 2001, p. 77). The report sidesteps the issue of which determinant trumps in a conflict by providing an example of compromise: Physicians are not expected to satisfy patients' demands for nonbeneficial treatment but are expected to respect informed refusal of beneficial therapy (Institute of Medicine 2001).

It is not difficult to translate the tension between an objective determinant of quality and a subjective one into the tension between beneficence and autonomy in the ethical domain. Nor should we be surprised if the conflict, which forms the basis of many ethical dilemmas in medicine, finds its way into the heart of the quality of care discussion. But the discussion of quality of care does not end with beneficence and autonomy. It includes fidelity, justice, and truth telling and begins to sketch the outline for a new ethic of professionalism. Indeed, the American College of Physicians in its recent charter on medical professionalism explicitly names commitment to improving quality of care as a professional responsibility (ABIM Foundation ACP-ASIM Foundation and European Federation of Internal Medicine 2002). Doctors now must not only do good but also do better.

The Quality of Health Care in Rural Practice

A quality chasm divides rural and nonrural areas, with equity or access to health care the primary cause (see chaps. 5 and 7). Despite technological advances and a growing physician pool, rural areas remain resource poor (Hart et al. 2002; Merwin et al. 2003; Bull et al. 2001). The promise of telemedicine (Marcin et al. 2004) has yet to be realized on any large scale, and rural physicians must often provide a larger scope of services than they would in a nonrural area. In certain areas, rural practice does not offer the volume necessary to either determine quality or to satisfy evidence-based notions of minimum standards for physicians to maintain competency.

While creative strategies have been devised to address or contest these issues (Allen and DeSimone 2002), the problem is more than "should this one physician be doing this procedure in this setting?" Rural health systems are fragile ecosystems. Recruiting and retaining personnel is difficult even in the best of times. Raising the bar of conformity to a fixed set of practice guidelines or limiting the scope of practice based on numbers can have detrimental effects that reverberate throughout the system, particularly if they negatively affect a marginal bottom line. In the extreme, the financial viability and existence of a rural institution may depend on its capture of the local market. Diverting services elsewhere may mean its demise, leaving the community severely or even completely unserved. Maintaining these services locally may mean that individual patients will receive less than optimal care, although the community as a whole will benefit.

Professional Roles

Ethical dilemmas in rural medicine have been attributed to close-knit relationships in rural communities where personal and professional relationships overlap and where physicians may have multiple social roles (Purtilo and Sorrell 1986; Roberts et al. 1999; see chaps. 2, 5, and 7). These same relationships affect what happens not only between physicians and their patients but also between physicians and their colleagues and physicians and the institution where they work (especially if it is also their employer). Referral patterns outside the local community do not go unnoticed in a setting where medical staff interactions resemble an extended family rather than a professional organization. For the individual physician, the ethical issues often boil down to loyalty to the individual patient versus loyalty to the institution that is the community's source of medical care.

Consider the following cases involving quality-of-care issues that illustrate the types of dilemma experienced by practicing rural physicians:

1. The generalist as specialist

Green County Hospital has a longstanding tradition of obstetrical care being offered by specialists and generalists, with routine deliveries being performed by family practitioners or obstetricians and Caesarian sections being performed by obstetricians or general surgeons. As demographics and physician training have changed, the obstetric cohort now consists of two family practitioners, a solo obstetrician, and an aging general surgeon. The surgeon's recently recruited junior partner has never performed a C-section but is willing to be trained and take call until a second obstetrician can be hired. He enters a preceptor arrangement with the obstetrician with the understanding that he will be credentialed by the institution when the obstetrician certifies that he is capable. His credentialing is fast-tracked after he performs a minimal number of procedures assisted by the obstetrician when a health crisis forces the retirement of the elder surgeon. The medical staff and hospital administration endorse the obstetrician's recommendation for privileges in spite of questions raised by one physician about the number of Caesarian deliveries successfully performed. Shortly after the surgeon receives C-section privileges, the obstetrician announces plans to leave on family business for two weeks.

One of the family practitioners doing deliveries feels ethically challenged by the situation. He appreciates the surgeon's overall competence but shares his colleague's reservation about the surgeon's ability to perform Caesarian deliveries. He will also be potentially involved in the surgery as assistant and will share the burden of any problems that may occur. He is concerned about his ethical obligations to his patients. He is also concerned about the fragile state of the surgical and obstetrical services at the hospital. Recruitment for both has been difficult, and decisions by either physician to leave now could collapse both services.

He knows that the obstetrician offers elective induction to his term patients before he departs on vacation and turns the service over to the surgeon. As a generalist, he had never felt the need to discuss the obstetrician's absence with his patients because the previous surgeon had a wealth of obstetric experience and had delivered babies for years. He consults with his family practice colleagues doing obstetrics about their ethical responsibilities to their patients. Neither has performed a C-section, although both have assisted on numerous occasions. One is less concerned and trusts that the obstetrician would not leave patients in incompetent hands during his absence. She likens the situation to their own training in larger institutions where they did procedures unsupervised after several successful attempts. She feels her colleague is carrying his obligation of nonmaleficence too far and that the requirements of truth telling do not include disclosure about the number of procedures done. She also reminds him of the larger issue of responsibility to the community, which has suffered the lack of consistent obstetrical services in recent years and now faces similar problems with surgery following the retirement of the last of its older generation of surgeons.

2. Securing scarce resources / adding new services

Far Plains Hospital has spent several months actively recruiting a second general surgeon to replace Dr. Smith, who was forced into early retirement. The hospital finds a well-trained, highly competent, midcareer surgeon with ties to rural life who would like to return to small-town life. Dr. Martin is, as far as anyone can tell, a good match for the practice she will share and for the community. Dr. Martin brings with her an interest in vascular surgery and experience with sufficient volume and excellent results. She wishes to continue with this surgery in her new location. Dr. Smith has had some training in vascular surgery, but his practice at Far Plains has been pretty much limited to the semiannual ruptured aortic aneurysm who will not survive transport or the occasional severed artery in a motor vehicle or farm accident. Dr. Smith welcomes the additional expertise and expanded service.

The hospital realizes that it will need to make a significant investment in equipment and personnel training to make the new service available. This will put the hospital's budget into the red but will result in future increased revenues that will offset the deficit. This investment will also provide some stability to the surgical service, which has been chaotic since the older partner was taken ill. The hospital hires Dr. Martin and commits to a vascular service.

The initial elective vascular surgeries are textbook successes. However, within a few months, there is an apparent increase in complications and morbidity in vascular patients. The complications are multiple and cannot be traced to a common source; the morbidity is not insignificant but not major. Dr. Martin's nonvascular patients are not involved in similar complications. Dr. Martin and the hospital have been rigorous in attempting to discover the problem(s) underlying the seemingly unrelated complications. Staff members have undergone additional training, the procedures and equipment have been examined and reexamined, and the affected patients' charts have been reviewed. Surgeries have been delayed pending the evaluation but are now ready to proceed in the absence of any clear-cut deficiency and with additional safety procedures in place.

Dr. Jones, a family practitioner, has been impressed with Dr. Martin and her forthright manner in dealing with the complications that have plagued her vascular service. Dr. Jones's patients who have undergone nonvascular surgery with Dr. Martin have done extremely well and have been happy with her services. To date, Dr. Jones has had no patients who have had vascular surgery at Far Plains. Dr. Jones's one referral to the surgeon for an aneurysm repair had his surgery postponed and is now scheduled for next week. He is waiting in Dr. Jones's exam room to review his medical clearance for surgery.

Dr. Jones is unclear about his ethical obligation to discuss the problems on the vascular service with his patient. In a previous job setting at a suburban hospital, such problems in the surgical department would remain largely unknown outside the department and would be blips on a background of much larger numbers. They would also be without such bottom-line importance to the hospital. This knowledge creates a tension between Dr. Jones's loyalty to the hospital, which is trying to do good for the community, and his loyalty to his patient, who may want to know why his surgery was postponed and whether he should have his procedure done at Far Plains.

Dr. Jones remembers the long and arduous effort to recruit the current surgeon, which began well before Dr. Smith's illness became critical. He remembers the chaos of having a temporary surgeon and the uneven care that was provided. Dr. Jones is aware that the current surgeon's agreement to come to the community was contingent on her ability to do vascular surgery. Dr. Jones does not wish to subvert the vascular service. But he knows that the patient waiting to see him is likely to ask: "Doc, if I was your mother, would you tell me to have my operation here?"

3. Subordinating community standards to community services

South Valley Regional Hospital serves an extended population of 25,000, offering mammography services that include state-of-the-art imaging and ultrasound backup. The hospital has invested heavily in its mammography suite and takes pride in providing local diagnosis and surgical treatment, including breast conservation surgery and sentinel node biopsy.

The mammography service is run by the solo hospital radiologist, Dr. Gray, who is meticulous in reading the films and is committed to early detection. Her diagnostic recommendation for suspicious microcalcifications or other abnormalities is excisional biopsy, an operative procedure, although other less-invasive options are available outside the local community. Her recommendations have resulted in a significantly higher incidence of breast biopsies being performed at South Valley than elsewhere in the state, but they also have led to the detection of a higher percentage of early cancers that is of unclear significance. Dr. Gray maintains that her approach offers the most definitive diagnosis and points to the statistics as demonstrating improved detection and earlier treatment. She also feels a strong commitment to maintaining services in the community and sees referral outside the community as a betrayal to the local hospital.

Family Practice of South Valley maintains a commitment to informed consent in patient care. Before referring its patients for surgery, the practice discusses options, including referral for procedures available at the tertiary care center (more than 100 miles away). In general this approach has worked to the benefit of the community, encouraging the surgeons to upgrade their skills or refer elsewhere for less-invasive procedures. With referrals for second opinions and needle biopsies generated by abnormal mammograms read by Dr. Gray, the process has backfired more often than not. Patients who choose options other than excision and return to South Valley for follow-up mammograms often find that Dr. Gray continues to recommend excision despite documentation of biopsy or stability of the abnormality. Frustrated patients often feel bullied or scared into subsequent biopsies. Angry ones choose to make an annual trip to the tertiary center for their mammograms.

Repeated episodes of such unhappy outcomes have forced Family Practice of South Valley to reconsider its informed consent discussion regarding abnormal mammograms. At least one member feels that the discussion should focus on the choice of local surgeon, discussing other options only if the patient brings up the issue. He argues that the present practice is resulting in more harm than good to the local community as well as to specific patients. Another member argues that informed consent is an obligation and not an option that can be sacrificed when inconvenient. At a minimum, she feels the group should offer to discuss other treatments with patients, especially when these treatments are mainstream medicine and offered in all large communities with dedicated breast centers.

4. Maintaining competence in critical services

Red Mountain Hospital is a 30-bed facility along the northern U.S. border. The hospital has always had an aggressive, competent medical staff interested in pursuing high-level care and serving the community well. The hospital has always maintained a small but fairly state-of-the-art ICU/CCU with trained and certified nursing and respiratory therapy staff. Throughout the years, the medical staff has had various discussions about critically ill patients and which ones were best served in the local community and which should be transferred to the tertiary care center. The decision was fairly obvious when the patient either specifically requested or adamantly refused transfer, needed services such as dialysis or a pacemaker that were not available at Red Mountain, or was imminently dying and not likely to survive transfer. Under other circumstances, the decision to stay or transfer was made by individual physicians and their patients/families, taking into account such factors as the intensity and anticipated length of critical care services, the comfort level and competence of the attending physician, and the ability to provide needed ancillary services. More aggressive physicians with greater critical care experience might choose to treat sicker patients locally than their counterparts.

Despite the coming and going of various physician members, the mix of the overall medical staff over the years has managed to support an adequate volume of ICU/CCU patients to maintain the competence of the service. This delicate balance has been threatened in the past few years as changing practices in the treatment of acute coronary conditions has resulted in earlier transfer for interventional procedures, namely cardiac catheterization, angioplasty, and stenting. For years, thrombolysis, the use of clot-busting medication, had been the mainstay of care for patients with acute heart attacks at Red Mountain. Depending on the response to therapy, these patients might remain at Red Mountain for their entire treatment and recovery period or be transferred to the tertiary hospital because of complications or for further evaluation, usually cardiac catheterization. An alternative therapy for heart attacks, primary intervention with angioplasty, was not an option because patients could not be transferred to the tertiary center in the required time.

This situation changed with the development of a protocol for acceler-
ated intervention in which heart attack patients were treated with modi-
fied thrombolysis in Red Mountain's ER and then immediately transferred
to the tertiary care center for intervention on arrival there. While aware
that this process would affect the CCU admissions, Red Mountain physicians endorsed it as a way of providing their patients with earlier intervention and better outcomes. Experience with the procedure, however,
forced them to reconsider their decision. Patients transferred from Red
Mountain did not always receive the intended intervention on arrival at
the tertiary center. Some waited a day or two. Some were discharged without it. Nurses tending the Red Mountain ICU/CCU with its low cardiac
census complained of the lack of ongoing coronary care experience.
Accompanying the acute patients during transport was not seen as a satisfying substitute because it lacked the structured safety of the hospital
environment.

The level of dissatisfaction triggered a medical staff meeting to review
the situation and its impact on Red Mountain Hospital and the community it serves. The discussion focused on the pragmatic issues of identifying the low-risk patients who received delayed intervention or no intervention and defining the benefits and harms to them, if any, of transfer to
the tertiary care center versus staying at Red Mountain. However, underlying the discussion was the tension between the need to maintain a competent critical care unit for the community and the desire to serve the best
medical interests of each individual patient. The level of discourse did not
rise to a discussion of theories of justice, nor did it fall to discussions of
economic impact. One practitioner, describing the dilemma, said: "How
can we provide the care we are expected to provide when needed, if we
are deprived of the experience necessary to maintain our skills?"

Good Enough

These four cases share contextual features. Each involves duties of
fidelity and/or truth telling to individual patients in situations regarding
treatment options. Each illustrates the ethical tension rural physicians
face in balancing their loyalty to an individual patient who may not receive the "best" care in a specific situation with their loyalty to the struggling institution that provides current and future care to this individual
and his community. Each is made more difficult by a lack of clarity in the

actual risks to the patient: How many C-sections does a competent general surgeon need to perform before being credentialed? What does the surgeon bringing a new technique or service to the community have to change before one is willing to say there is no increased risk? How does a physician determine which critically ill patients will have an increased survival benefit from tertiary care?

While one could draw analogies between the duties of the physicians in these situations and the duties of physicians in managed care or other aggregate settings where there is a conflict of loyalties (Emanuel 2000; Wolf 1994), these comparisons would not adequately address the situation of rural physicians. The rural hospital is not an impersonal insurer attempting to limit care and maximize profit. Rather, it is the sometimes heavily mortgaged medical home to the community and its practitioners that depends on the support of those it serves. This community relationship is morally relevant. However, there is still the need to disclose to patients information important to helping them make medical decisions. But such social relationships among rural institutions, practitioners, and the community may necessarily shape the process or content of disclosure. As H. Tristram Englehardt notes in *The Foundations of Bioethics,* "The more patients and physicians share a common view of the goals of health care in particular and of life in general, the less necessary elaborate disclosures need be. However, some disclosures will always be necessary. Friends need to know, even if only implicitly, the character of their joint endeavors" (1996, p. 297). Perhaps, the rural situation is not so different from, "What would you do (or tell) your mother, Doc?"

Rural physicians and their patients have always struggled with issues of quality of care. When either physicians or patients have felt sufficiently compromised, referral out of the community, now described as rural bypass (Radcliff et al. 2003), was the chosen option. How many careers or health care services have been negatively affected in the process will never be known. Likewise, the implications for the health of those communities affected will never truly be known.

As quality of care becomes a professional and political imperative, rural physicians must be able to grasp the relevant ethical dimensions of their roles as providers of care to populations that are geographically isolated, often poor, and desirous of a medical home that provides services when needed in the community. Standards applicable in the world of the well staffed and well supplied may not always apply. There is the desirable, and there is the possible. In the world of the rural physician, the question often is: "Is the possible good enough for my patient?" The ethical dimensions of the question and how it is answered remain a dilemma for the rural physician.

REFERENCES

ABIM Foundation, ACP–ASIM Foundation, and European Federation of Internal Medicine. 2002. Medical professionalism in the new millennium: A physician charter. *Annals of Internal Medicine* 136 (3): 243–46.

Allen, J. W., and K. J. DeSimone. 2002. Valid peer review for surgeons working in small hospitals. *American Journal of Surgery* 184 (1): 16–18.

Bull, C. N., J. A. Krout, E. Rathbone-McCuan, and M. J. Shreffler. 2001. Access and issues of equity in remote/rural areas. *Journal of Rural Health* 17 (4): 356–59.

Calico, F. W., C. D. Dillard, I. Moscovice, and M. K. Wakefield. 2003. A framework and action agenda for quality improvement in rural health care. *Journal of Rural Health* 19 (3): 226–32.

Emanuel, E. J. 2000. Justice and managed care: Four principles for the just allocation of health care resources. *Hastings Center Report* 30 (3): 8.

Engelhardt, H. T. 1996. *The foundations of bioethics.* New York: Oxford University Press.

Gifford, F. 1996. Outcomes research and practice guidelines. Upstream issues for downstream users. *Hastings Center Report* 26 (2): 38–44.

Grol, R. 2001. Improving the quality of medical care: Building bridges among professional pride, payer profit, and patient satisfaction. *Journal of the American Medical Association* 286 (20): 2578–85.

Hart, L. G., E. Salsberg, D. M. Phillips, and D. M. Lishner. 2002. Rural health care providers in the United States. *Journal of Rural Health* 18 Suppl:211–32.

Hofer, T. P., R. A. Hayward, S. Greenfield, E. H. Wagner, S. H. Kaplan, and W. G. Manning. 1999. The unreliability of individual physician "report cards" for assessing the costs and quality of care of a chronic disease. *Journal of the American Medical Association* 281 (22): 2098–105.

Institute of Medicine. 2001. *Crossing the quality chasm: A new health system for the 21st century.* Washington, DC: National Academy Press.

Marcin, J. P., J. Ellis, R. Mawis, E. Nagrampa, T. S. Nesbitt, and R. J. Dimand. 2004. Using telemedicine to provide pediatric subspecialty care to children with special health care needs in an underserved rural community. *Journal of Pediatrics* 113 (1): 1–6.

Merwin, E., I. Hinton, B. Dembling, and S. Stern. 2003. Shortages of rural mental health professionals. *Archives of Psychiatric Nursing* 17 (1): 42–51.

Purtilo, R., and J. Sorrell. 1986. The ethical dilemmas of a rural physician. *Hastings Center Report* 16 (4): 24–28.

Radcliff, T. A., M. Brasure, I. S. Moscovice, and J. T. Stensland. 2003. Understanding rural hospital bypass behavior. *Journal of Rural Health* 19 (3): 252–59.

Roberts, L. W., J. Battaglia, M. Smithpeter, and R. S. Epstein. 1999. An office on Main Street: Health care dilemmas in small communities. *Hastings Center Report* 29 (4): 28–37.

Rosenblatt, R. A. 2002. Quality of care in the rural context: A proposed research agenda. *Journal of Rural Health* 18 Suppl:176–85.

Stirrat, G. M. 2004. Ethics and evidence based surgery. *Journal of Medical Ethics* 30 (2): 160–65.

Wolf, S. 1994. Health care reform and the future of physician ethics. *Hastings Center Report* 24 (2): 28–41.

CHAPTER 9

Building Bioethics Networks in Rural States

Blessings and Barriers

FRANK CHESSA, PH.D., AND JULIEN S. MURPHY, PH.D.

Access to resources in bioethics is important to quality patient care. Rural states, however, confront significant challenges in developing and sustaining resources in bioethics. In urban areas, bioethical expertise typically disseminates from major medical centers with large training programs. But in rural states, major medical centers are less common. Further, labor-intensive bioethical resources, such as an ethics consultation service, are rarely self funding and thus require a large institutional infrastructure for support. The fiscal resources may simply not be available in small rural clinics or in the potentially overburdened medical centers in rural states that service the needs of the rural poor. A further challenge is that only one or a few individuals in a rural community are likely to have training in bioethics, and thus the resources are fragile as organizations built around their expertise may collapse should one or more crucial members become unable to participate.

In addition to these challenges, the types of ethical issues facing rural health care providers may differ from those facing urban providers. Several articles suggest that the close-knit nature of rural communities raises issues of confidentiality, surrogate decision making, and the provider-patient relationship in ways that are specific to rural communities (Cook and Joyner 2001; Glover 2001; Kelly 2003). Thus, training and reference materials developed in urban settings may be less likely to help with the ethical issues that arise in rural communities. While rural health care workers may be just as earnest as their urban counterparts about acting in their patients' best interests, they may find few, if any, bioethical resources available or relevant to their practice (see chaps. 2 and 7).

Building a statewide bioethics network is a good strategy to meet the needs of rural states. Indeed, practitioners in some rural states have built networks, and several of these networks have met with success, fulfilling the need for bioethics resources among practitioners in rural states. However, for every successful network, there are multiple failed attempts and multiple networks that are minimally active and that struggle to survive. The literature on rural bioethics, which is thin in all topic areas, is virtually silent on networks. There is no data on the factors that influence the success or failure of attempts to establish ethics networks in rural states. Indeed, as far as we know, there is no resource that catalogs bioethics networks. Similarly lacking is a national bioethics network organization to provide resources and leadership to regional networks. The American Society for Bioethics and the Humanities (ASBH), the leading professional interdisciplinary organization in the field, offers sessions on rural ethics at its annual conference, and these meetings have provided support for building and sustaining rural networks. For instance, this chapter was first presented at an ASBH conference, and an Illinois network also credits the ASBH for its beginnings (Anderson-Shaw 2006).

We begin this chapter by investigating the theoretical underpinnings of the concepts "bioethics" and "rural," which frame our inquiry. A tempting assumption is that the types of bioethics resources and knowledge that are useful to practitioners in urban settings would be equally useful in rural settings. Indeed, as educators in rural states, we have in the past adopted this assumption ourselves, insofar as we used concepts and curricula developed in urban settings for trainings presented at rural hospitals and clinics. However, when we examine the assumption critically, it does not hold true. Later, we turn our attention to clarifying the idea of a rural bioethics network. What we uncover in the conceptual exercise of defining a rural bioethics network is that a definition with a narrow focus on rural ethics excludes most existing bioethics networks from counting as a *rural* bioethics network. Thus, as a practical matter of making bioethics expertise available to rural communities, we focus not on rural bioethics networks but on bioethics networks in rural states. We provide a case study of one such network—the Maine Bioethics Network. While in many ways the network's character is unique to Maine, the case yields lessons for the sustainability and role of a bioethics network that services rural states. The section called "Establishing a Rural Bioethics Network" addresses issues in the development and sustenance of rural bioethics networks. We conclude by evaluating the blessings and barriers these networks present in meeting the bioethics needs of rural areas.

Establishing Rural Bioethics

Rural bioethics is emerging as a small but important niche within the burgeoning field of bioethics. To date, there has been virtually no research on health care ethics in rural settings. A recent literature survey identified only 55 articles on rural health care ethics in more than three decades (Nelson and Weeks 2006; Nelson et al. 2006). Those interested in rural bioethics may find the relatively small number of articles discouraging, but the attention William Nelson and colleagues have paid to rural bioethics is encouraging. That a study was designed to cull through several large medical and interdisciplinary databases in search of articles in bioethics with a rural focus attests to the emergence of rural bioethics as a new niche in the field of bioethics. Most of the articles Nelson and his colleagues identified were descriptive rather than offering new normative principles or theory for bioethics in rural settings. Further, commentators on Nelson noted that his search criteria might themselves reflect an urban bias in that rural practitioners writing about issues in their practices might not use the nomenclature of urban bioethics, even though the issues they uncover are "ethical issues," broadly construed (Cook and Hoas 2006; Hardwig 2006; Miller 2006; see chaps. 7 and 8). These observations suggest the need for original research that is sensitive to the language and the distinctive ethical issues in rural health—the sort of research begun by Ann Cook and her colleagues at the National Rural Bioethics Project at the University of Montana (Cook and Hoas 2000; Cook, Hoas, and Joyner 2000; see chap. 3).

A second aspect of creating rural bioethics as a subfield or niche is defining it. In a recent issue of the *American Journal of Bioethics*, commentators discussed how rural contexts offer different perspectives on the provider/patient relationship and the role of community, among other issues (Fryer-Edwards 2006; Klugman 2006; see chap. 1). The commentator consensus is that we need to pay more attention to rural bioethics. Rural bioethics research will likely expose the erroneous assumption, identified by Jessica Miller (2006), that rural communities are homogenous or monolithic. In addition, journals need to be receptive to issues in rural health as well as rural ethics. We have found only one journal that has an exclusively rural focus, the *Journal of Rural Health.*

A third aspect of establishing rural bioethics is to identify rural practitioners and relevant texts. Recently, an analysis of members of the ASBH found that only 2 percent of the membership lived or worked in a rural setting (Nelson and Weeks 2006; see chap. 2). This finding indicates that rural health care is typically isolated from national bioethics resources. Ethics consultation services, the mainstay for urban bioethicists in hospital settings, are not typically found in rural settings. Small hospitals in rural states usually lack full-time or even part-time ethicists. Of the 40 hospitals in Maine, only one hospital has a full-time ethicist—that is, a staff member devoted exclusively to ethics consultation and education— and this position is a recent development. Other hospitals in Maine rely on medical staff with interest in bioethics to serve on clinical ethics committees and to provide leadership on ethics in the areas of research and policy. Nurses and physicians are often self taught in clinical ethics. Rural content is also lacking in bioethics textbooks for university students and health professionals, even on rural campuses. The transferability of content to rural contexts that is generated from urban contexts is assumed though untested.

Undeniably, the field of bioethics has been dominated by the concerns and values of urban health care providers. John Hardwig has remarked that bioethics is "an urban phenomenon" (2006, p. 53). Narratives of the history of bioethics are also urban in character. The history of the field typically finds the midwives of bioethics to be attending to concerns related to emerging technologies in large medical centers (e.g., dialysis machines, ventilators, genetics, in vitro fertilization) (Jonsen 1998; Stevens 2000). Although there are important exceptions to this trend—for example, Craig Klugman (2006) points out that the Tuskegee study, a classic in research ethics, was both low-tech and conducted on the rural poor—the narratives of the urban birth of bioethics prevail nonetheless. A technological focus, particularly the implications of new technology— which usually is available only in urban settings—on patient care is a main theme in the bioethics literature.

The growing awareness of biases in bioethics, such as its urban focus, is useful for the further development of the field. To understand the limitations of a profession opens up a critical space to explore its objectives and scope and to ask new questions—such as those about potential racial biases in the field (Myser 2003). One new question concerns the nature of rural bioethics: Is American bioethics inextricably urban, such that rural concerns will always be derivative or subordinate? This conjecture seems likely given recent changes in health care delivery in rural areas. Hardwig (2006) suggests that the niche of rural bioethics might be emerging too late if health care is vanishing from rural America. He notes the closures of small hospitals. While small hospitals are shutting down, new quick-care clinics are opening up. If this trend continues, rural health care may come to mean nonspecialty care provided by walk-in clinics. Patients with acute needs would be transported to urban medical centers. The concerns of rural bioethics would be radically altered in the absence or significant downsizing of rural health care delivery. Measures to provide support to rural bioethicists need to be flexible to adjust to the changing landscape of rural health care. Rural bioethics networks can go a long way to providing a forum for discussing trends in rural health care, including the privileging of urban centers for subspecialty care. As Lisa Anderson-Shaw (2006) notes, networks contribute to research by first bringing together rural providers to identify and discuss rural health care needs.

Rural Bioethics Networks

Like much of what emerges in rural settings, bioethics networks are cobbled together from available resources. Rural bioethics networks vary in mission, objectives, design, organizational structure, and funding sources. Lacking a national model for rural networks makes describing these varied, often improvised, structures challenging. We begin by identifying the core features of a rural bioethics network, and then we lay out some of the various forms that such groups do and potentially can take.

Our working definition of a rural bioethics network is a confederation of clinicians, administrators, academics, and others interested in health care ethics who communicate with one another in an effort to learn about the ethical issues that arise in the provision of quality health care in rural communities and to provide resources and support to those working in health care in rural areas.

According to our definition, a rural bioethics network has two core functions: (1) to learn about ethical issues in health care in rural communities, and (2) to provide resources and support to health care workers in rural areas (see chap. 12). Both criteria must be understood loosely. "Learning" can take the form of reviewing literature, case discussions, or sponsoring a research study. "Resources and support" can be the type of support that a practitioner in a rural community would gain by taking part in a case discussion, as well as Web sites, newsletters, speakers' bureaus, curricula, conferences, and policy discussions, to name a few. The definition is also loose in other ways. There is no requirement that members be exclusively or even primarily from a rural setting, nor is there a requirement that the network be based or physically located in a rural setting. In addition, our definition prioritizes interest in bioethics over formal training. There is no requirement that members of a network have ethics training through graduate courses or certificate programs. The network may provide informal training through reading groups, journal clubs, brown bag lunches, or by sponsoring ethics lectures.

What sorts of organization does the definition exclude? First, "network" carries the connotation that the group's membership not be contained within the walls of one institution. Rather, "network" suggests that members come from a variety of settings and that there is a sharing of information among individuals from various settings. So, while a single institution may sponsor a network (i.e., provide financing, administration, communication technology, or space), members typically come from a variety of settings and institutions (e.g., hospitals, long-term care facilities, state public health agencies, colleges and universities, religious institutions, law firms, research institutes, etc.). Networks are not necessarily bioethics centers or institutes, although such entities may sponsor networks.

A second component of the definition is that such networks should be focused, at least in part, on rural communities. Thus, the network must consider ethical issues likely to arise in a rural community as well as provide services to those working in rural communities (see chap. 2). Because the resources in rural bioethics are so sparse, some networks may export standard bioethical educational resources to rural practitioners in order to critically examine the relevance of these materials for the issues and problems that arise in a particular rural community. Rural practitioners may also be interested to know about trends in urban ethics literature, not only because patients move between rural and urban health care settings but also because practitioners want to examine urban research from a rural

perspective. Other networks study bioethical issues that arise in rural settings but do not provide resources back to such communities. Still other
networks may aim to generate new rural resources. Given that resources
are limited in rural areas, rural bioethics networks, in some cases, may
depend for their survival on collaborations with urban bioethics centers
and institutions. Rural bioethics networks that receive financial and in-
kind support from an urban institution, and draw members largely from
urban institutions, take care to ensure that rural members set the agenda
of meetings and suggest the cases or issues discussed. Networks that function as urban-rural hybrids balance the interests of both groups and, in
some cases, may have rural subgroups that focus exclusively on rural
issues. The importance of a good working relationship between urban and
rural members of a network cannot be overstated. Resources may largely
or at least initially come from urban areas such as larger hospitals or colleges that provide medical training and outreach to rural communities.
Urban members of rural networks can be important partners with rural
providers. After all, some urban providers and educators daily transverse
the urban/rural divide as they care for rural patients, train rural chaplains
in city hospitals, or educate rural nurses in city colleges.

Assuming that the above definition captures the core characteristics
of rural bioethics networks, the next reasonable question to ask is: How
many entities meet the above definition? Rural networks lack national
visibility and are difficult to count. Like other rural activities, some networks will use the Internet as a vital tool for their members. None of the
bioethics networks serving, in part, rural communities are exclusively
rural in focus or name. Our Internet survey identified six bioethics networks in North America with Web sites: the Canadian Bioethics Network,
the Florida Bioethics Network, the Bioethics Network of Ohio, the Pied-
mont Bioethics Network in North Carolina, the Virginia Bioethics Network, and our own, the Maine Bioethics Network. Three rural bioethics
activities are explicitly linked to public universities: For example, the
Nevada Center for Ethics and Health Policy located at the University of
Nevada, Reno, has a subgroup focusing on rural health. Rural bioethics is
a specific focus of the Center for Bioethics and Humanities at the University of Colorado at Denver, and the National Rural Bioethics Project is located at the University of Montana.

Why are there so few easily identifiable bioethics networks? We present
a case study to provide some insight into this question and others. We

discuss how one bioethics network emerged, thrived, faltered, and was redesigned, all within little more than a decade of existence.

Case Study of a Rural Bioethics Network

Cases play an important role in bioethics. Sometimes the legal, academic, and public reactions to a single case are the primary factors that result in new national policy. To cite one example, guidelines regarding withdrawing artificial nutrition and hydration emerged almost entirely from the Nancy Cruzan case, and there has been little change in them since then. A case study narrative also keeps scholars attached to the concrete problems of real people—discussions of bioethics theory do not often highlight the pain, indecision, and heartbreak of persons who find themselves in a real-life bioethical dilemma. Finally, using cases in bioethics typically involves attending to the unique features and rich detail of each case. Even while general lessons emerge from cases, so does an understanding of how a dilemma faced by an individual clinician emerges in a particular form because of its unique social and historical context. Contextualization is a valuable aspect of the case study methodology because it allows a questioning of assumptions that are largely invisible until the social and historical context is given explicit attention.

Here we offer a case study of the Maine Bioethics Network (MBN). The case study is useful for examining networks in rural states for several reasons. First, Maine has much in common with other rural states, and so the factors in Maine that give rise to the perceived need for a network, as well as the challenges to building a network, are likely to be similar to those of other states. Identifying and analyzing commonalities among rural states can help us develop collective strategies for networks across rural states. We also learn from our differences, and so we highlight some of the unique features of Maine and the MBN. The story of the development of the MBN is interesting in itself, but one of the purposes of highlighting the uniqueness of Maine is to remind ourselves that every rural community is multifaceted and unique. Our impression is that some rural communities have exceptionally strong collective identities. This distinctiveness is bound to influence how community members feel about the bioethical issues arising in that community. For example, Kelly Fryer-Edwards (2006) describes a radio program in a small town in Wyoming that weekly reads a list of the in-patients at its community hospital, and how HIPAA regulations brought an unwelcome change to the community by forcing an end to this activity. By contrast, in rural communities in the Northeast, for instance, where notions of Yankee privacy and decorum continue to thrive, we could not imagine community support for the public airing of a list of hospitalized individuals.

As members of the MBN board, we have been directly involved with the history of the organization over the past several years. This expertise puts us in a good position to know some of the inner workings of the organization. Of course, this participation also means that we do not write with a detached, objective attitude. Although we strive for accuracy, we are not unemotional about the history and fate of the MBN. We claim no impartiality in the study. We are invested in and committed to the success of the MBN, wanting to identify and act in the best interests of the board and members in its role of service to the state.

Maine is primarily a rural state. The population of 1,321,505 (in 2005) is dispersed throughout sixteen counties over 30,000 square miles, for a population density of 40 persons per square mile (State of Maine 2006). Portland, Maine's largest city, has a population well under 100,000 (State of Maine 2006). There is a seven-campus public university system, as well as a number of private colleges, one law school, one osteopathic medical school, several nursing programs, and a few graduate programs. Few large companies or businesses call the state home. The largest employer is a health insurance company, Unum Provident, with 13,000 employees, and the second-largest employer is a public hospital, the Maine Medical Center, with 5,000 employees (Career One Stop 2007). Maine is a relatively poor state and struggles with relatively low rankings on a number of socioeconomic measures. The average household income in Maine is $42,500 (35th of 50 states) (U.S. Census Bureau 2006). Maine has had a poverty rate of between 10 and 12 percent since 1994, with the highest poverty rate of 21 percent in Washington County (its most northern county) (Maine State Planning Office 2005). One-third of the citizens have income at or below the 200 percent of the poverty level, an index used to measure income necessary to provide for the basic needs of a family of three (Maine State Planning Office 2005), and 17 percent of children under age five are below the poverty line (Maine State Planning Office 2005). Maine is 96.9 percent Caucasian, making it the state with the highest percentage of whites. Maine's most prominent culture is French-Canadian—many Mainers speak both French and English, and French-Canadian social clubs are

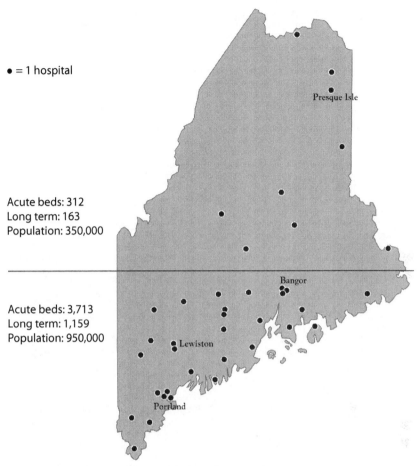

• = 1 hospital

Acute beds: 312
Long term: 163
Population: 350,000

Acute beds: 3,713
Long term: 1,159
Population: 950,000

Figure 9.1. Distribution of hospital beds in the state of Maine
Source: Adapted from the Maine Hospital Association with permission.

common. Recently, Maine has become a primary and secondary resettle-
ment area for immigrants from Somalia and other African countries. Portland also has thriving Korean and Vietnamese communities.

If one divided the surface area of Maine roughly in half geographically
by drawing a horizontal line fifteen miles north of Bangor, 75 percent of
its population would fall below the line in the southern half of Maine (see
Figure 9.1) (Maine Hospital Association 2003). Maine's four largest population centers (Portland, Lewiston/Auburn, Waterville, and Bangor) are all
south of the line, as are almost all of Maine's colleges and universities and
the majority of its tourist industry. These differences are also reflected in

health care resources. Of Maine's 40 hospitals, 34 are in the southern half, as are 37,000 of its 40,000 acute-care beds and 1,150 of its 1,400 long-term care beds. While the state has roughly the national average of acute-care beds per capita (2.6 per 1,000 residents in Maine, 2.7 nationally), it has only ten beds per 100 square miles, compared to a national average of 20 and a New England average of 51 (Maine Hospital Association 2003). The data suggest, and our anecdotal experience supports this, that persons with complex health care needs in the northern half of the state must travel at least as far as Bangor (more than four hours), and probably much further south, to receive in-patient specialty care.

The MBN was established in 1994 in part because of burgeoning interest in Maine in the death-with-dignity movement. As a founding member recalls, three large conferences were scheduled for the same day, all of which devoted significant time to ethical issues in death and dying. Both sponsors and participants at the conferences quickly realized that coordinating bioethics activities in the state would be beneficial. Among the founding members were faculty members from the University of New England, Bates College, and the Bangor Theological Institute, an obstetrician, a health care attorney, a medical sociologist from an independent research institute, a leader in the Maine Nurses Association, and a leader of the Maine Council of Churches.

The new network developed three objectives: education, outreach, and networking. Its stated goals were to provide forums for exploring values, rights, and responsibilities that should underlie the health care system; to promote collaborations and communications among its members and other individuals and groups on bioethical issues; and to serve as an educational resource for professionals, the public, and policy makers. The network's aim was to be a statewide organization that would be nonpartisan and nonprofit. The MBN was incorporated as a 501(c)(3) corporation with a set of bylaws that recognized two categories of members—individuals and institutions. The primary source of funding was and continues to be membership dues and donations. The bylaws established a board of directors but entrusted the membership at large with voting privileges for most major decisions. Voting on major issues has taken place at an annual meeting of members. At its peak in 1999, the MBN had 280 members. Many hospitals purchased an institutional membership, which allowed staff to attend meetings and educational programs.

The difficulties in sustaining a rural network are illustrated by the un-

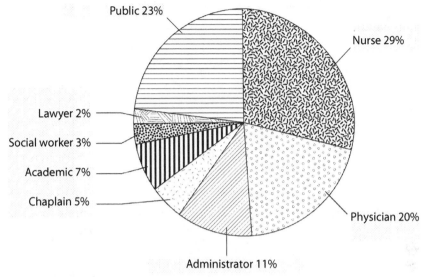

Figure 9.2. 1999 MBN membership, by profession

even development of the network. For this discussion, we have divided the history of the MBN into three phases.

Phase I: 1994–2000

The first six years of the network were its most successful. The network held annual member conferences and sponsored continuing education programs at professional conferences. During this period of time, the MBN received administrative support from an association representing assisted living, nursing home, and other long-term care facilities in Maine. In addition to this tie to long-term care facilities, 16 of Maine's hospitals joined the MBN. Figure 9.2 provides information on the professions of members.

During this phase, the MBN decided to maintain a neutral position on policy issues, providing open and balanced forums for discussion. This decision was significant because from 1998 until 2000, Maine was the primary battleground in the national physician-assisted suicide debate. After the practice was legalized in Oregon in 1997, Maine was thought to be the next state that would legalize it. Despite strong early support, the referendum was defeated in the popular vote (51% to 49%). Our interviews with past members inevitably turn to the role the MBN played in this debate. Public interest in bioethics was at an all-time high in Maine. MBN meetings in 1999 were not quiet affairs in which professionals discussed esoteric issues in their field of expertise. Instead, members viewed themselves as taking part in a vigorous public discussion that ultimately would influence the important step Maine would take regarding physician-assisted dying.

Phase II: 2000–2004

In its middle years, the network suffered a number of problems. The professional association that had been providing administrative support had to stop providing this support, leading to financial difficulties for MBN. There was a leadership vacuum and no consensus on its mission. Some members wanted to expand the scope of the organization, build its membership, and vigorously fund-raise. Others were skeptical about increasing staffing needs for such an ambitious direction. During this period, collecting dues from members became difficult. Indeed, dues had always been little more than a charitable contribution on the part of individuals and institutions because MBN programs were offered to the public for free or at a minimal charge. As a small organization, we were unable to negotiate price breaks on bioethics journals or other membership benefits. There was debate among board members about whether corporate sponsorship was appropriate, though this option was not pursued. Members also voiced concern about housing the network within one institution, rather than receiving support from a statewide association. Given these debates, as well as a general scarcity of offers to provide administrative support, the MBN was not able to find a stable administrative home. Administrative tasks were divided among several members of the board working at different organizations. The MBN board president and officers were unpaid, and these positions floated among a number of individuals. The lack of consistent leadership and administrative support led to an inability to expand membership or raise money. The MBN came to have an increasingly inactive membership and uneven participation from the board. In part, this was due to geographical constraints. As a statewide organization, the board was committed to holding its meetings in a central location. However, that required several hours of driving for most board members. Participation in board meetings, given the transportation time, was a significant time commitment. In addition, many board members were playing several leadership roles in their own communities and institutions, thus affording little time for long travel commitments.

In Maine, as is probably the case in other rural states, interest in bioethics is sustained by a small number of "champions" whose professional roles, more likely than not, do not include formal responsibilities or compensation for participating in bioethics-related activities. During this time, the organization suffered the death of its president, a physician who had been involved in end-of-life care and was actively leading the organization. Shortly thereafter, a longstanding board member, also a physician with expertise in ethics, suddenly died. Two unexpected deaths on the board within fifteen months were catastrophic for the network. As in large urban centers, those with interest and training in ethics in rural areas are typically serving on many committees at the workplace and also may participate in key roles in community organizations. However, in rural states, there may be few people equipped to replace key members. For a few years, the MBN board grappled unsuccessfully with these issues. The board finally voted to place the organization in an inactive state with the intention of rebuilding the board and reinvigorating the network after a brief hiatus.

However, even during this relatively unstable period, the MBN was able to sponsor three statewide conferences and numerous educational sessions at Maine health care conferences. Individual members from different geographical areas and work settings continued to network with one another and in large part considered the MBN to be a vital place for those who work in isolation at their respective institutions to come together to discuss ethical issues with others who shared the same interests. An interesting partnership in this regard is the connection between academics and clinicians. Academics (notably philosophy and theology professors) found it valuable to speak with the clinicians who have daily contact with "real" patients and the technical expertise necessary to understand the medical details of national cases. Similarly, clinicians without formal training in ethics found it valuable to interact with professionals who could lay out, with no hesitancy, the intellectual puzzles in ethics that arise, for example, from the distinction between killing and allowing to die. Persons from a variety of backgrounds participated in discussions, but the clinician-academic partnership was important in sustaining the

energy of the organization. While the value of a partnership between philosophers and clinicians is not limited to rural settings, a network is one
of the few ways to make such a partnership possible in rural states.

Phase III: 2004 to the Present

Since 2004, new members of the board have brought the MBN out of
dormancy and reorganized so that the network provides a useful resource
to professionals interested in bioethics. The first problem to solve was
finding support from an institution. Primarily, the network was in need of
some infrastructure, such as support staff and Web page support. In selecting a suitable organization, the board wished to continue an unbiased
perspective (e.g., not an insurance company) and to be statewide (e.g., not
a specific hospital). One model considered was that of an academic journal housed at a university for a fixed time period and rotating among
universities over time. One university was seen as a good choice, in part
because it was not hospital-affiliated and a board member had just established a bioethics center there, which would give visibility to the network.
Thus, the Maine Bioethics Network is now housed at the University of
Southern Maine (USM), though the resources USM can provide are limited. New persons were added to the board, with an attempt to include
persons from around the state. The board is considering a model that
would be a constellation of satellite groups from the north, south, and
central regions of the state. This clustering would allow for regional meetings and activities, and each satellite would be connected to the larger
network. MBN has sponsored a well-attended public forum on the Terri
Schiavo case, continuing education for social workers, and "lunch and
learn" meetings for board members and other interested persons. There
has been a good deal of interest in MBN; professionals moving into the
state have sought it out as a forum for discussing bioethical issues, and
longtime members still consider MBN to be the place where such discussions occur in Maine.

Resources in bioethics in Maine have continued to grow with the hir-
ing of a full-time ethicist at the Maine Medical Center, the state's largest
hospital. Moreover, ethics committees at the larger hospitals in Lewiston
and Bangor are becoming more active, in part because of the influence of
staff newly trained in bioethics affiliated with these institutions. There
are a number of health care ethics conferences in the state, and most peo-

ple working in bioethics in the state know one another and correspond regularly.

The primary barriers to an active network are Maine's geography and the busy lives of local persons interested in bioethics. After several years of trying a frontal assault on these barriers by the traditional means of organizing meetings at convenient locations and dates, and meeting with little success, the board is relying on the Internet to establish a virtual network of members. There will be no dues to belong to the network, and indeed "membership" will have much less meaning as the electronic resources will be open to everyone. The MBN will have less emphasis on statewide meetings. Instead, the hope is to use a Web site and listserv to link persons in Maine working in bioethics.

Two issues are of concern in this transformative process. First, members of the MBN in its first stages identified with being a member of the organization. Indeed, in our experience, a surprising number of people identify themselves as founding members of the organization and exhibit pride in their role in sustaining the organization. It will be interesting to observe whether downplaying the importance of membership in the organization will negatively affect loyalty to the MBN. Second, most persons who are currently active professionally are already likely to access Internet resources such as Bioethics.net, which features the *American Journal of Bioethics,* national news articles, and a blog. The use of Google to research questions is widespread, and many subscribe to national e-mail newsletters and listservs. However, the ease of accessing national information in the field is not matched with quick access to local information, issues, and discussions. People are likely to value learning about the conference that is in the next city, or within an hour's drive, and is therefore easy to attend. But, will there be a commonality of experience about bioethical issues within Maine that will make it especially useful for Mainers to talk among themselves about the issues? Or, is a health care provider in rural Maine just as likely to find an understanding ear and sage advice from someone in Nevada or Mississippi or New York City for that matter? The ability of the MBN to sustain itself, even as a virtual network, will likely depend on how these issues play out.

Establishing a Rural Bioethics Network

Establishing networks of any type can be challenging in rural settings. Rural areas, even when rich in natural resources (e.g., farmland, mining, forestry, fisheries), can be depleted in economic resources. There may be little infrastructure for rural nonprofit organizations. The idea of establishing a bioethics network may arise in rural communities, but frequently it emerges in urban settings, such as professional bioethics conferences or discussions among faculty on college campuses. The Illinois Health Care Ethics Forum, which Anderson-Shaw (2006) describes, emerged from an ASBH conference, and the MBN originated from discussions within a private Maine university and is currently affiliated with a public urban university. Many networks emerge from and are sustained by urban resources for good reasons. Urban ethicists can be important allies of their rural counterparts when they recognize the needs of rural areas and marshal some resources to this end. Sometimes alliances between urban and rural ethicists emerge from common experience, when urban ethicists have grown up in or lived and worked for a time in rural areas or when rural ethicists have previously lived in large cities or worked for large health care institutions. Remembering our own experiences living in rural areas can quickly teach us the importance of quality rural health care and the need for the field of bioethics to include a rural focus.

In our case study above, we identified various issues related to the network's mission, organizational structure, objectives, financial support, leadership, and staffing. In addition, there were geographical issues, such as how to build viable connections between many small, relatively isolated communities hours apart. The organizational structure of rural networks will vary as will rural contexts. We have learned several lessons from our experience in Maine. Chief among them is the value of linking a network to other organizations with related interests. A network is a web of relationships, and the bigger the web, the more points of connection, the more people involved, and the more resources one can expend. The mission of a rural bioethics network needs to meet the internal needs of network participants or external needs of the region, or both. Each group that gathers to build a network needs to consider the unique issues of network participants and the pressing bioethics questions in the region. The aim of a network may be simply to share information and provide support for health care providers across a region, or it may focus on community education or address pending health care policy issues. A network may emerge or for a time be sustained by a single issue that demands attention because of local concerns, for instance, improving end-of-life care, addressing health care rationing, or providing insight into proposed abortion restrictions. Other networks may find that the level of training in ethics is a common need. If so, networks need to critically evaluate the kinds of training available, taking into account online programs if members cannot travel, tapping local resources, or supporting efforts for some members to pursue summer ethics training programs. Networks emerge easily when there is a cohort of interested, enthusiastic people who work well together. Sustaining leadership over the years can be difficult if the network does not also continually develop and encourage the talents and interests of longtime as well as new members.

When working with few resources, it is easy to worry about success. What counts as success for a rural network must be thought about critically. Each rural bioethics network must define success on its own terms in light of its own goals. Thus, each group will need to determine criteria for measuring its own success. Goals must be realistic and must take into account the competing demands on members from multiple professional and personal roles. The goals must include some issues that members care about deeply, as well as ones that the network can reasonably expect to accomplish. This may include ecological activities. A network may wish to join with environmental groups to address the connections between environmental degradation and local health issues (e.g., living downwind of the peppermill or next to the landfill) or issues of rural poverty (e.g., rates of asthma, diabetes, obesity, or smoking-related illnesses) or issues of social justice (e.g., the problem of the uninsured or, for those with some sort of coverage, the high cost of prescription drugs). A long view can be helpful in assessing any grassroots organization, and rural networks are no exception. Markers of success may vary from network to network, and it will usually be unrealistic to apply urban achievements to rural contexts. Even if a network is struggling or small or does not reach the entire designated area, it may be successful simply by being a community benefit. After all, little things can matter a great deal in our daily practices.

Sustaining a rural network can be as challenging as establishing one. While some aspects of small towns (distance from high crime rates, high cost of living, and the traffic of big cities) are treasured by rural residents, other aspects present barriers for network building. Sustaining a network can be difficult when resources are scarce, infrastructure nonexistent, and the number of people with ethics training to develop the network few. But even when progress is slow, we have found many blessings in our involvement with MBN. First, the network brings together those who share a deep interest in bioethics. Second, networks provide valuable support for practitioners, providers, theorists, educators, and interested members of the public. One of the genuine limitations of rural living is its isolation. A network is an important antidote to this. It also offers resources that might not otherwise be found. For instance, if the network is statewide, it allows members to have a state perspective, to understand how problems differ or may be the same from region to region, and in many cases, it provides members with contact from people in other regions of the state that they would not otherwise have had. Networking is critical in a rural state where the few people trained in ethics are scattered throughout a large geographical region and there is no medical school at the center of ethics training. The network is a necessity, not a luxury, for staying informed and helping one another with ethical issues that arise in clinical practice.

Persons who wish to establish a network will have to consider the resources and barriers specific to their location and target audience. However, some general tactics about beginning a network have emerged from our experience and research, and these may be useful to others beginning a network:

- Identify a core planning group to develop initial goals and objectives.
- Identify sources of financial and institutional support in the region.
- Consider local and state issues that might help to develop interest among persons in your state.
- Develop a communication plan for networking members across geographic areas early in the process—do not allow the initial interest of new members to wane for lack of contact from the network.
- Develop a schedule of activities early in the process—sustain the interest of new members or those at a "kickoff" event by allowing them to put into their calendars upcoming events sponsored by the network.

Likewise, we also offer the following potentially helpful list of guidelines for sustaining a network:

- Identify dedicated people who have the time, talent, and interest to sustain the network.
- Develop a template of activities and set of expectations around leadership positions so that potential leaders know how much time the position requires and so that new leaders do not have to "reinvent the wheel."
- Develop a meeting schedule for the board (and perhaps for the general membership) and stick to it.
- Evaluate financial resources and institutional support: Are they adequate for the programmatic objectives of the network? Are they potentially alienating to some members of the target audience?
- Consider public events for outreach and membership building.
- Partner with other professional groups in the state.
- Plan events that match the needs of members and the region.

We believe in the importance of bioethics networks in rural areas. As our definition of a rural bioethics network states, the goal of the network is to support health care practitioners in providing good-quality health care in rural settings. People living in rural areas have the same right to good-quality health care as those in urban areas. Networks are an important resource for rural providers, from advocating for rural community hospitals as employers and care providers, to allowing family members to be cared for near their homes where they can easily be visited by family and friends, to advocating for more rural practitioners. Bioethics networks in rural areas can help communities and health care providers learn the language of morality in order to provide excellent care and to be advocates for their own existence on a larger stage. In all these ways, networks can be an important contributor to good-quality rural health care.

NOTE

We would like to thank Richard Gelwick, Ph.D., for discussing the origins of the Maine Bioethics Network and Susan Stark, Ph.D., for offering helpful comments on an earlier draft.

REFERENCES

Anderson-Shaw, L. 2006. Rural health care ethics: What assumptions and attitudes should drive the research? *American Journal of Bioethics* 6 (2): 61–62.

Career One Stop. 2007. State of Maine: Largest employers. America's CareerInfo-Net. www.careerinfonet.org/oview6.asp?soccode=&stfips=23&from=State&id=11&nodeid=12 (accessed January 15, 2007).

Cook, A. F., and H. Hoas. 2000. Where the rubber hits the road: Implications for organizational and clinical ethics in rural healthcare settings. *HEC Forum* 12 (4): 331–40.

———. 2006. Re-framing the question: What do we really want to know about rural healthcare ethics? *American Journal of Bioethics* 6 (2): 51–53.

Cook, A. F., H. Hoas, and J. C. Joyner. 2000. Ethics and the rural nurse: A research study of problems, values, and needs. *Journal of Nursing Law* 7 (1): 41–53.

Cook, A. F., and J. C. Joyner. 2001. No secrets on Main Street. *American Journal of Nursing* 101 (8): 67, 69–71.

Fryer-Edwards, K. 2006. On cattle and casseroles. *American Journal of Bioethics* 6 (2): 55–56.

Glover, J. J. 2001. Rural bioethical issues of the elderly: How do they differ from urban ones? *Journal of Rural Health* 17 (4): 332–35.

Hardwig, J. 2006. Rural health care ethics: What assumptions and attitudes should drive the research? *American Journal of Bioethics* 6 (2): 53–54.

Jonsen, A. 1998. *The birth of bioethics.* New York: Oxford University Press.

Kelly, S. E. 2003. Bioethics and rural health: Theorizing place, space, and subjects. *Social Science and Medicine* 56 (11): 2277–88.

Klugman, C. M. 2006. Haves and have nots. *American Journal of Bioethics* 6 (2): 63–64.

Maine Hospital Association. 2003. Interesting facts about Maine's hospitals. www.themha.org/members/hospitalfacts.htm (accessed January 15, 2007).

Maine State Planning Office. 2005. 2005 report card on poverty. www.maine.gov/spo/economics/economics/pdf/povertyreport2005.pdf (accessed January 2007).

Miller, J. P. 2006. Defining "research" in rural healthcare ethics. *American Journal of Bioethics* 6 (2): 59–61.

Myser, C. 2003. Differences from somewhere: The normativity of whiteness in bioethics in the United States. *American Journal of Bioethics* 3 (2): 1–11.

Nelson, W., G. Lushkov, A. Pomerantz, and W. B. Weeks. 2006. Rural health care ethics: Is there a literature? *American Journal of Bioethics* 6 (2): 44–50.

Nelson, W., and W. B. Weeks. 2006. Rural and non-rural differences in membership of the American Society of Bioethics and Humanities. *Journal of Medical Ethics* 32 (7): 411–13.

State of Maine. 2006. Facts about Maine. www.maine.gov/portal/facts_history/facts.html (accessed January 2007).

Stevens, M. L. T. 2000. *Bioethics in America: Origins and Cultural Politics*. Baltimore: Johns Hopkins University Press.

U.S. Census Bureau. 2006. 2005 data. www.census.gov/hhes/www/income/income05/ (accessed January 2007).

CHAPTER 10

Structural Violence in the Rural Context

The Ethical Implications of Welfare Reform for Rural Health

ELIZABETH A. THOMAS, R.N.C., PH.D., M.P.H.

Passage of the 1996 Personal Responsibility and Work Opportunity Reconciliation Act (PRWORA) restructured the welfare system in the United States and radically changed the way the federal government and states assist poor women with children. This chapter examines the ethical implications of the reformed welfare system as it affects rural women, using the concept of structural violence as a theoretical framework to critically assess the ethical issues embedded in contemporary rural workfare realities. An examination of the ethical issues of rural welfare is a necessary precursor to health care policy reform and further program development aimed at improving rural health outcomes and building rural communities. Health care program development requires a critical analysis of how the implementation of present workfare requirements, when levied against rural women, can create a social system with an undercurrent of structural violence, an insidiously destructive social fallout that may further erode rural health.

With the enactment of PRWORA, welfare changed from the open-ended entitlement program of Aid to Families with Dependent Children to the temporary assistance program, Temporary Aid to Needy Families (TANF). Social scientists, health care providers, economists, and other professionals representing a cross-section of disciplines have identified that PRWORA instituted a profound social change with long-term economic, health, and social consequences that are only now being fully realized (Findels et al. 2001; Kneipp 2000a; Kneipp 2000b; Rural Policy Research Institute 1999; Taylor 2001; Weber, Duncan, and Whitener 2001; Whitener 2005; Whitener, Gibbs, and Kusmin 2003). PRWORA changed the federal government's 60-year history of guaranteed cash assistance for poor women and replaced it with a block grant governed by the states that limits welfare enrollment and includes mandatory work requirements, establishment of paternity, and special living arrangement requirements for teen parents (Taylor 2001). According to the Rural Policy Research Institute, welfare reform shifted the "philosophy of welfare from hardship alleviation to employment and in doing so focused the processes within welfare to connecting individuals with appropriate skills to economic opportunities" (Rural Policy Research Institute 1999, p. 11). This change signaled a philosophical shift in government's response to poverty in the United States. Women raising children were now required to become self-sufficient wage earners and financially support their own children. TANF tied support to compliance with outside-of-the-home work.

The effect of PRWORA on rural populations, particularly women, is of considerable concern for health care providers and public health planners. Women in rural communities are being held to the same standards as their urban-living counterparts, but by the nature of their rural living status, they are less able to stay in compliance with work requirements. The rural context holds substantial social, economic, and geographic barriers to finding and maintaining employment. All health care providers need to understand how the welfare system itself has the potential to diminish health and even inflict injury. Physicians and nurses working in rural areas and those working in urban, tertiary referral health care facilities need to be aware that the contemporary welfare system may impede health promotion programs and exacerbate health disparities.

To gain a more in-depth understanding of the interrelatedness of rural living, welfare, and women's health, nurse educators, nurse researchers, and practicing nurse clinicians will need to join with public health and social scientists to examine the ethical implications of any social system that undercuts women's health. The cumulative burden of attending mandatory work seminars, training programs, and workfare placement appointments, combined with failing or fragile local economies, and geographic isolation exacerbated by inadequate or nonexistent public transportation has created a social service system that further stresses the already pronounced physical and psychosocial stress of poor rural women.

An Ecological Approach

A critical analysis of the ethics of welfare reform in rural populations requires using an ecological perspective, a perspective that provides the theoretical foundation to explain how the interactions of persons with their most immediate social environment (the micro- and mesosystems of family and community), the more distant exosystems of region, state, and country, and the macrosystems of socioeconomics, politics, and culture are all intertwined.

Urie Brofenbrenner (1979) brought ecological theory to the attention of social scientists and the health care disciplines, conceptualizing human development as emerging from the interaction of the individual and a multilayered, intertwined social environment. He views the environment as a series of nested, sequentially larger, and more encompassing levels of social context. He explains that a person's perceptions form through reflection, challenges, and demands to cope with and adapt to the overall social environment.

According to Robert A. Hahn (1995), illness is an individual's subjective experience of lacking health. Nancy Krieger (2001) describes the science community's current understanding of illness and disability as having evolved beyond the traditional models of the host-agent-environment triad and a linear chain of events toward a more ecological perspective that is multidimensional and dynamic. The focus of an ecological perspective is determining what are the driving forces behind the changing patterns of social inequalities in health (Krieger 2001). Michael Agar (2003) urges the health care community to adopt qualitative epidemiology, a theoretical merging of ecological theory and complexity theory, to employ a "person-in-context" conceptualization of health and illness, a perspective that embraces both historicity and place. Neil Pearce stresses the importance of examining the context in depth when looking at the cause of diseases in populations, noting "it is essential to understand the historical and social context and to emphasize the importance of diversity and local knowledge rather than looking for universal relationships" (1996, p. 682). In other words, context and individual experience matters.

Defining Structural Violence

When health care providers and policy makers employ an ecological perspective to examine social systems, they allow for a wider focus, moving away from public interventions targeting individual behavioral change toward a more encompassing consideration of those macrosystems that alter societal contexts and have the ability to generate and perpetuate structural violence (Lane et al. 2004). Identifying how the intersections of social, political, economic, and cultural factors can create structural dysfunction and violence in social systems is a critical step in improving the health of rural people.

The conceptual framework of structural violence was first described by Johan Galtung as a part of his work in peace research. Galtung states, "violence is present when human beings are being influenced so that their actual somatic and mental realizations are below their potential realizations" (1969, p. 168). Galtung used the epidemiological concept of the potential as a way to define violence, identifying that violence as "the cause of the difference between the potential and the actual, between what could have been and what is . . . violence is that which increases the distance between the potential and the actual, and that which impedes the decrease of this distance, . . . when the potential is higher than the actual it is by definition avoidable and when it is avoidable, then violence is present" (1969, pp. 168–69).

Galtung describes "violence as avoidable insults to basic human needs, and more generally to life, lowering the real level of needs satisfaction below what is potentially possible" (1990, p. 292). He designed a typology of direct and structural violence, describing how direct violence and structural violence influence the four basic needs (survival needs, well-being needs, identity/meaning needs, and freedom needs). Galtung stated that structural violence is a process of exploitation or unequal exchange and may be viewed as a permanent part of the culture (1990, p. 294).

The avoidable distance between the potential health and well-being and the actual condition of health and oppression is a central element of structural violence. In his work examining structural violence in global populations using population theory methodologies, Tord Hoivik (1977) explains that the definition of structural violence is based on the gap between the actual and potential conditions, a concept that is half-empirical and half-theoretical, noting that the actual world can be observed and measured, but the potential can only be conjectured or modeled. Hoivik emphasizes that "structural violence measures the distance between an actual society and a potential one, one without structures of violence" and requires the use of demographic theory and population theory concepts to design models that can help social scientists envision the shape and scope of structural violence (1997, p. 60).

Reflecting Galtung's and Hoivik's conceptualization of structural violence as a gap between the actual and potential, Deborah Du Nan Winter and Dana Leighton (2001) narrow the definition of structural violence to any constraint on human potential caused by embedded economic, legal, and political structures and cultural traditions. David G. Gil focuses on the nature of structural violence, defining it as "violence in human relations [that] is rooted in socially evolved and institutionalized inequalities of status, right and power among individuals, sexes, ages, classes and peoples" (1986, p. 124). Susan E. James and colleagues note that violence "stems from, and is legitimatized by, situations of oppression . . . [and that] violence is a subset of oppression" (2003, p. 129). Conceptualized structural violence is different from other types of violence because it is subtly embedded within society (James et al. 2003). James and colleagues describe structural violence as being "built into the fabric of society based on norms and traditions that subjugate one group in favor of another" (2003, p. 130) and assert that a major characteristic of structural violence is that its consequences affect one group differently from another and are disseminated through the mechanisms of the state and its social institution. Gil echoes social inequality as the essential element of structural violence, noting that "social-structure violence" may itself be considered a "consequence of inegalitarian social structures" (1986, p. 127).

In this chapter, structural violence is defined as the destructive consequence of a social system that is characterized by a type of oppression and inequality of power and rights according to gender, race, age, and class that is embedded in the fabric of society. Structural violence tends to lead to social inequality and vice versa, creating a vicious cycle.

Contemporary Cases

The unintended negative, destructive consequences of social policy and political agendas are often seen most dramatically in society's poorest populations. James and colleagues state, "the most visible indicators of structural violence are the differential rates of mortality, morbidity and incarceration among groups in the same society" (2003, p. 130). Paul Farmer, a physician and medical anthropologist, identifies the world's poor as "the chief victims of structural violence and [they] are not only more likely to suffer; but they are also less likely to have their suffering noticed . . . suffering is differentially weighted in different settings" (2003, p. 50). Farmer (1996, 1999a, 1999b, 2003, 2004) has extensively analyzed the connection of poverty to the occurrence of death and illness worldwide. He examines the problem in depth in *Infections and Inequalities: The Modern Plagues* (1999b) and more recently in *Pathologies of Power: Health, Human Rights, and the New War on the Poor* (2003). In both texts, using specific case studies in real-world settings, Farmer argues that political agendas, global economic upheaval, rural population displacement, rural-to-urban migration, and racial, ethnic, and gender discrimination create the intractable poverty that drastically heightens rural people's vulnerability to disease, disability, and death. For example, Farmer describes how political repression and the economy-driven displacement of farmers to less arable land directly increased the spread of AIDS in rural Haiti because it led to further impoverishment of Haitian farmers and subjected rural Haitians (mostly women) to sexual exploitation when forced to travel to urban areas to find work. Farmer's extensive analysis of the spread of AIDS in Haiti provides a clear example of how interconnected rural poverty is with the occurrence and outcome of disease.

Consistent with Farmer's analyses of how the macrosystem and social injustice contribute to disability and disease, many contemporary sociologists, psychologists, and public health professionals are encouraging researchers and policy makers to consider individual behaviors within the larger context of social, political, economic, and cultural systems. John B. McKinlay and Lisa D. Marceau (2000) propose a hierarchical approach to examine how the layering of social structure, environment, and lifestyle makes an impact on physiology and results in the occurrence of disease. Terry C. Pellmar, Edward N. Brandt, and Macarn A. Baird (2002) propose that a concept of allostatic load may be used to examine the interference of sociopolitical processes in health. They describe allostatic load as overwhelmed physiologic systems, such as stress-related disorders. Ronald M. Andersen, in the most recent revision of the Behavioral Model of Health, includes the external environment (including physical, political, and economic components) as "an important input for understanding health services" (1995, p. 6).

Structural Violence and Rurality

Despite a growing awareness of an ecological perspective, many health care providers have little or no understanding about the life-course stress of rural patients. Few physicians and nurses comprehend how structural violence in the sociopolitical system of welfare affects the health of rural patients. Even health care providers living in small rural communities may have never driven in the poor part of town or witnessed (let alone experienced) the tedium, frustration, stigmatization, and humiliation of standing in the food stamp or unemployment line. To develop a fully informed ecological perspective about the experiences of rural welfare recipients, one must examine the rural context.

Sociopolitical structural violence is the most powerful form of structural violence because the state has the ability to exercise legal authority (James et al. 2003). Persistent lack of (or withholding of) information and extensive surveillance systems are two common types of sociopolitical structural oppression that poor rural women experience. Information (especially the need to provide it when demanded) itself is a prominent type of oppression for poor rural women. Acquiring and keeping all the necessary paperwork (rent leases, utility bills, job interview verifications, doctor excuse slips when missing work) becomes a time-consuming undertaking made often more difficult in rurality by the distance required to go to various offices and get the papers needed.

Rural women who are migrants experience an additional burden—fear of deportation. When migrant women attempt to enroll in welfare and Medicaid, the welfare system's demand for information may be a distinct form of oppression, as these women may be further victimized because they are either unable (or afraid) to provide the necessary information and documentation to complete the application. Lastly, the disclosure of private information and loss of privacy required to apply for and comply with welfare create a type of destruction of self-worth. Pamela A. Monroe and Vicky V. Tiller (2001) note that the lack of anonymity and the stigma of poverty and being welfare reliant are powerful factors limiting TANF participation and contribute to the emotional and psychological stress of the welfare-reliant in rural Louisiana.

In a three-year investigation, Susan Hays explored the experience of women on welfare. Her findings are chronicled in her book *Flat Broke with Children: Women in the Age of Welfare* (2003b). Hays witnessed the surveillance burden (her terms) that mandatory seminars, training programs, and workfare placements placed on welfare mothers. She notes that in many cases women who failed to attend job-readiness or employment-training sessions or failed to report a sufficient number of job contacts were sanctioned.

Hays (2003b) describes sanctioning as a form of punishment for failing to comply with welfare rules, and it means that all or parts of the welfare benefits are cut. Sanctioning is a graduated process in most states and can result in being permanently ineligible for welfare benefits. Funds are cut during sanctioning, but the welfare clock continues running, using up the lifetime allotment of benefits. Sanctioning offenses include failure to make job contracts, attend scheduled meetings with caseworkers, attend job-readiness classes, arrive on time at the workplace, cooperate with child support enforcement, as well as getting fired for a workplace mistake or quitting a job without proving "good cause." Personal illness or a child's illness are not counted as "good cause" (2003b). In the description of sanctioning consequences, Hays provides an example of sociopolitical violence, stating that when "sanctioned welfare clients lost all or part of their family's welfare for a specified number of months—they lost, in other words, their primary source of income" (2003a, p. B8). Hays states that roughly one-quarter of welfare recipients are sanctioned or denied benefits for failure to comply with welfare rules (2003b).

The Rural Policy Research Institute (RUPRI) (1999) argues that successful welfare reform must connect persons having the appropriate job skills to economic opportunities, but rural people are less likely to have the needed job skills due to fewer years of formal education completed and lack of available job training. Rural areas also provide limited job opportunities because these areas are dominated by limited base economies, seasonal work, and industries or service sector jobs that pay low salaries. The RUPRI reports rural workers are more likely to earn minimum wage and be underemployed. The persistent depression of rural salaries lowers tax revenues and reduces the likelihood that rural areas can retain higher-skilled laborers and attract new businesses. Many rural families remain poor even when workers are fully employed (Whitener, Gibbs, and Kusmin 2003).

Rural Geography and Economics

The geography of rurality contributes to and intensifies poverty. A key characteristic of the geography of rurality is distance. Distance contributes to the most significant rural barriers to getting a job and staying employed: the lack of childcare, transportation, health care, and housing (Findels et al. 2001; Rural Policy Research Institute 1999; Weber, Duncan, and Whitener 2001). Remoteness imposes a barrier because distance has real economic costs in terms of money and time spent in traveling from place to place. Due to their low population densities, rural areas have too few childcare providers, while available providers offer limited slots and usually restrict service to daytime hours. Geographic isolation, lack of public transportation, and dependence on private vehicles to reach distant worksites further intensify the burden of mandatory work requirements and job training meetings.

The geography of rural areas, characterized by distance, complicates every aspect of working for a rural woman raising children. In many rural areas, school consolidation has profoundly increased the distance between home, school, and work. Taking a child to the babysitter or picking up a sick child from school may require a roundtrip of well over two hours even when a reliable vehicle is available. The increased cost of gasoline further limits a poor woman's ability to find and keep a job that is usually offering only minimum wage. The lack of reliable childcare combined with the lack of transportation contributes to the emotional stress and fear of sanctioning. Hays identifies that a system of enforced work in a context that undermines the work of poor women does not even make sense economically: "The federal support of paid childcare for the poor makes obvious one of the central cost-benefit contradictions in the logic of welfare reform. The costs of subsidizing childcare for the poor far outstrips the state and federal costs of paying a welfare mother to raise her own children. It is cheaper, by far, to give a mother her monthly welfare check than it is to subsidize her childcare at market rates" (2003b, pp. 71–72).

Redesigning Welfare

The current welfare system itself contributes to a culture of structural violence. To redesign the welfare system and dismantle destructive policies, policy makers must develop a more thorough understanding of the rural context and what the experience of being welfare reliant in rural communities entails. Current state and federal policies need to be critically examined to determine how they negatively affect the rural welfare-reliant woman's ability to comply. States will need to develop region-specific rural strategies as a part of their TANF plans. Policy makers, health care providers, rural communities, and welfare recipients must come together to determine what are the most critical needs for their state's rural welfare-reliant population. States will need to develop processes and procedures that prevent the need for sanctioning. Expanding work-related activities, case management support, brokering services, transportation, and child-care support are some of the strategies needed to reduce the structural violence of welfare sanctioning (Bloom and Winstead 2002; Kaplan 1999, 2004).

To create an effective, empowering welfare system, research is needed that takes a macrosystem, ecological perspective in viewing the rural environment. Farmer calls for a new research agenda that examines "the multiple dynamics of health and human rights, on the health effects of war and political-economic disruption, and on the pathogenic effects of social inequalities, including racism, gender inequality and the growing gap between rich and poor, [asking] by what mechanisms do such noxious events and processes become embodied as adverse health outcomes" (2003, p. 241). To legitimatize reforming welfare and better comprehend how the current welfare system policies make welfare compliance difficult, research agendas must include qualitative investigations that identify the issues and the system barriers as they are experienced by rural women on welfare. Farmer challenges health care professionals to listen to the voices of those on the receiving end of structural oppression, noting, "whether they are nearby or far away, we know, often enough, who they are" (1999a, p. 1492).

Health care professionals should consider how political agendas have shaped the policies, structures, and processes of the contemporary welfare system, creating an oppressive system for many of those enrolled. The ethics of demanding compliance, sanctioning noncompliance, and valuing only outside-the-home, paid work as a socially valid form of employment is called into question when the physical, economic, and social environment imposes structural barriers that actually impede compliance and limit outside-the-home job opportunities. Identifying the destructive system flaws in the current design and administration of PRWORA and revising the system to reflect the geographic, social, and economic realities of rural living will require a commitment to ongoing, collaborative work by all parties—rural communities, health care providers, public health planners, and public policy makers. The critical first step to end many of the oppressive structures of welfare reform is to recognize that the geography of rurality matters and to value the voices of the women trapped in a politically created culture of structural violence. We cannot afford to have the lived reality of rural women decided in out-of-touch legislative offices. What is merely a cost-and-benefit analysis to some is an untenable life for many. Reform is not a luxury but a necessity to save rural women from lives of structural violence.

REFERENCES

Agar, M. 2003. Toward a qualitative epidemiology. *Qualitative Health Research* 13 (7): 974–86.

Andersen, R. M. 1995. Revisiting the behavioral model and access to medical care: Does it matter? *Journal of Health and Social Behavior* 36 (1): 1–10.

Bloom, D., and D. Winstead. 2002. Sanctions and welfare reform. Brookings Institution. www.brookings.edu//papers/2002/01welfare_bloom.aspx (accessed August 24, 2004).

Bronfenbrenner, U. 1979. *The ecology of human development*. Cambridge, MA: Harvard University Press.

Farmer, P. 1996. On suffering and structural violence: A view from below (how poverty influences suffering). *Daedalus* 125 (1): 261–84.

———. 1999a. Pathologies of power: Rethinking health and human rights. *American Journal of Public Health* 89 (10): 1486–96.

———. 1999b. *Infections and inequalities: The modern plagues*. Berkeley and Los Angeles: University of California Press.

———. 2003. *Pathologies of power: Health, human rights and the new war on the poor*. Berkeley and Los Angeles: University of California Press.

———. 2004. An anthropology of structural violence. *Current Anthropology* 45 (3): 305–25.

Findels, J. L., M. Henry, T. A. Hirschl, W. Lewis, I. Ortega-Sanchez, E. Peine, and J. N. Zimmerman. 2001. *Welfare reform in rural America: A review of current research*. Columbia, MO: Rural Policy Research Institute.

Galtung, J. 1969. Violence, peace, and peace research. *Journal of Peace Research* 6 (3): 167–91.

———. 1990. Cultural violence. *Journal of Peace Research* 27 (3): 291–305.

Gil, D. G. 1986. Sociocultural aspects of domestic violence. In *Violence in the home: Interdisciplinary perspectives,* edited by M. Lystad. New York: Brunner/ Mazel.

Hahn, R. A. 1995. *Sickness and healing: An anthropological perspective.* New Haven, CT: Yale University Press.

Hays, S. 2003a. Studying the quagmire of welfare reform. *Chronicle of Higher Education,* October 17, B7–9.

———. 2003b. *Flat broke with children: Women in the age of welfare reform.* New York: Oxford University Press.

Hoivik, T. 1977. The demography of structural violence. *Journal of Peace Research* 14 (1): 59–73.

James, S. E., J. Johnson, C. Raghavan, T. Lemos, M. Barakett, and D. Woolis. 2003. The violent matrix: A study of structural, interpersonal, and intrapersonal violence among a sample of poor women. *American Journal of Community Psychology* 31 (1–2): 129–41.

Kaplan, J. 1999. The use of sanctions under TANF. *Welfare Information Network Issue Notes* 3 (3). The Finance Project. www.financeprojectinfo.org/all_pubs .cfm (accessed August 24, 2004).

———. 2004. Addressing the needs of adults sanctioned under TANF *Welfare Information Network Issue Notes* 8 (2). The Finance Project. www.financeproject info.org/all_pubs.cfm (accessed August 24, 2004).

Kneipp, S. M. 2000a. The health of women in transition from welfare to employment. *Western Journal of Nursing Research* 22 (6): 656–74; discussion 674–82.

Kneipp, S. 2000b. The consequences of welfare reform for women's health: Issues of concern for community health nursing. *Journal of Community Health Nursing* 17 (2): 65–73.

Krieger, N. 2001. Theories for social epidemiology in the 21st century: An ecosocial perspective. *International Journal of Epidemiology* 30 (4): 668–77.

Lane, S. D., R. A. Rubinstein, R. H. Keefe, N. Webster, D. A. Cibula, A. Rosenthal, and J. Dowdell. 2004. Structural violence and racial disparity in HIV transmission. *Journal of Health Care for the Poor and Underserved* 15 (3): 319–35.

McKinlay, J. B., and L. D. Marceau. 2000. To boldly go. *American Journal of Public Health* 90 (1): 25–33.

Monroe, P. A., and V. V. Tiller. 2001. Commitment to work among welfare-reliant women. *Journal of Marriage and Family* 63:816–28.

Pearce, N. 1996. Traditional epidemiology, modern epidemiology, and public health. *American Journal of Public Health* 86 (5): 678–83.

Pellmar, T. C., E. N. Brandt Jr., and M. A. Baird. 2002. Health and behavior: The interplay of biological, behavioral, and social influences: Summary of an Institute of Medicine report. *American Journal of Health Promotion* 16 (4): 206–19.

Rural Policy Research Institute. 1999. *Rural America and welfare Reform: An overview assessment.* Columbia, MO: Rural Policy Research Institute.

Taylor, L. C. 2001. Work attitudes, employment barriers, and mental health symptoms in a sample of rural welfare recipients. *American Journal of Community Psychology* 29 (3): 443–63.

Weber, B., Weber, B. A., G. J. Duncan, and L. A. Whitener. 2001. Where do we go from here? The impact of welfare reform on rural families and implications for the reauthorization debate: Welfare reform in rural America: What have we learned? *American Journal of Agricultural Economics* 83 (5): 1282–92.

Whitener, L. A. 2005. Policy options for a changing rural America. *Amber Waves* 3 (2): 28–35. U.S. Department of Agriculture Economic Research Service. www .ers.usda.gov/AmberWaves/April05/pdf/april05_feature_policyoptions.pdf (accessed December 19, 2006).

Whitener, L. A., R. Gibbs, and L. Kusmin. 2003. Rural Welfare Reform: Lessons Learned. *Amber Waves* 1 (3): 38–44. U.S. Department of Agriculture Economic Research Service. www.ers.usda.gov/Amberwaves/June03/pdf/awjune2003rural refromfeature.pdf (accessed August 18, 2004).

Winter, D. D. N., and D. C. Leighton. 2001. Structural violence. In *Peace, conflict and violence: Peace psychology for the 21st century,* edited by D. J. Christie, R. V. Wagner, and D. D. N. Winter. Upper Saddle River, NJ: Prentice Hall.

CHAPTER 11

Rural Geriatric Bioethics

A Texas Perspective

WILLIAM J. WINSLADE, PH.D., J.D., AND
MARTHA BEARD-DUNCAN, M.A., J.D.

Old Main Street office long time burn down. No [hometown]
doctor anymore. Only brand-new, sooperdooper Medical Center.
Too far away. But all doctor stay there together. I say, why need
so many doctor in same sooperdooper place? Better to spread
out, little doctor here, little doctor there. Better the old-fashioned
way.

Ozeki 1998, p. 156

This chapter presents some ideas about geriatric bioethics issues.
After providing background information about rural Texas health services
and typical medical problems of elderly people, we present an overview
of geriatric bioethics issues faced by rural Texans.

In terms of access to care, the rural elderly people of Texas are vastly
underserved. As Daniel Patrick Moynihan observed, "A commonplace of
political rhetoric has it that the quality of a civilization may be measured
by how it cares for its elderly" (1996). In terms of caring for rural elderly
people, Texas is not measuring up and needs to take steps to care for this
ever-growing demographic. As this chapter demonstrates, the senior citizens of rural Texas are a fragile lot. It may seem impossible to simply boost
the quantity of health care providers in rural Texas without significantly
increasing expenses. Treating the rural elderly people of Texas as well as
the urban elderly people requires the efficient use of public funds. Thus,
if one accepts the premise that all elderly people deserve to be treated

with equal dignity, no matter whether circumstances placed them in a wealthy Houston neighborhood or a fading border town, it follows that as the population ages, creative stopgap health care measures should be expanded and implemented.

The Health Care Landscape for Texas's Rural Elderly People

This section provides an overview of rural Texas, its elderly people, and the challenges they face in obtaining health care. These challenges include geographical isolation; the problems of providing access to health care in isolated, sparsely populated rural areas; shortages of medical professionals; the medical problems of rural elderly people; racial and cultural barriers; and a lack of insurance. Additionally, this section briefly examines the health care challenges faced by Texas inmates—an aging group, largely located in rural locales.

About Rural Texas

It is not easy to determine or to define *rural* as it applies to Texas.

Policymakers at the state and federal levels have long struggled with how to assess the rurality of a given geographic area. As of November 2002, there were 24 different definitions of "rural" in Texas statutes and the Texas Administrative Code. Similarly, three federal agencies each use different definitions that are applied by federal legislation to various health programs. According to the U.S. Census Bureau, 2,907,272 resided in "non-urban" Texas in 2000, while the White House Office of Management and Budget (OMB) designated 2,946,750 Texans as nonmetropolitan residents in 2003. In addition to these designations, the extreme isolation of many communities has given rise to a subset of rural and nonmetropolitan known as "frontier." The Department of Agriculture Economic Research Service (ERS) has classified 29 Texas counties as completely rural and not adjacent to a metropolitan area, while the National Rural Health Association has adopted a definition that classifies 131 Texas counties as frontier. (Eskridge 2004)

For our present purposes, however, it is sufficient to point out that as of 2003, 177 of 254 counties in Texas were classified as nonmetropolitan (Texas Department of Health Center for Health Statistics 2004). Despite the seeming dominance of nonmetropolitan counties, however, as of 2003 only 13.6 percent of Texans (approximately 3 million out of 22 million) resided in nonmetropolitan areas (Texas Department of Health Center for Health Statistics 2004). In contrast, before World War II most Texans lived on ranches, farms, or in rural communities (Murdock et al. 2000). Perhaps the most rural area of the state is far West Texas. Excluding the major city of El Paso, far West Texas can be classified as both a "border" and a "frontier" region.[1] The area consists of eight counties with a combined landmass of 30,500 square miles (U.S. Census Bureau 2007). Its total population is only about 54,000 people, or 2.4 percent of the Texas population (U.S. Census Bureau 2007). Other parts of Texas—such as South Texas, the Panhandle, or far East Texas are also sparsely populated, albeit less so than the deserts of far West Texas.[2]

Access to Health Care in Rural Areas in Texas

The sparse population and isolation of rural Texas give rise to what is perhaps the most significant bioethics issue for Texas's rural elderly population: access to health care (see chap. 1). Medical services of all kinds are limited in rural areas because of closing of community hospitals and reduction of emergency room services (Associated Press 2004; Valdez 2004). Where smaller communities do have hospitals, their diagnostic and technological capacities may be limited. In rural communities populated by ranchers and farmers, travel time to hospitals increases risks to seriously ill or injured persons. For example, a 59-year-old rancher in West Texas who initially concealed his dizziness and nausea lost consciousness and awoke in a pool of his own blood. He was taken to a local hospital, more than 30 miles from the rancher's home, but the staff could not diagnose his illness. He was promptly sent by helicopter more than 200 miles away. He was diagnosed there with an unusually severe case of diverticulitis. He had lost three units of blood. If he had had to wait any longer for transfusions, he probably would have gone into shock.

Even persons who are relatively close to an emergency room may not receive adequate attention for their medical needs. At the same emergency room mentioned above, a 70-year-old Hispanic woman who lived only a few miles from the hospital, after complaining of severe chest pains, was told that she would have to wait six hours before a physician could see her. Her response was, "If I'm going to die, I'd rather do it at home than here in the waiting room" (personal communication with Martha Beard-Duncan). Fortunately, she did not die and eventually saw a doctor who diagnosed her with acid reflux disease. This example raises several issues: Why was the rancher evaluated, referred, and transferred to an urban facility comparatively promptly? Could it have been related to the fact that his wife was an elected official and the rancher himself was a prominent citizen? Why was the elderly Hispanic woman not seen promptly? Was it because she was Hispanic or elderly or because the emergency room was overworked and understaffed? It is difficult to determine which explanation is correct, but in any case such discrepancies are a serious problem.

A Shortage of Medical Professionals

Rural areas of Texas have difficulty recruiting physicians and nurses even when there is a local hospital.[3] Compounding an already problematic situation, some commentators predict a growing nationwide shortage of physicians and nurses, especially those trained to care for America's aging population (American Geriatric Society's Core Writing Group of the Task Force on the Future of Geriatric Medicine 2005). The population of older adults is increasing in rural Texas (Texas Department on Aging, Office of Aging Policy 2003), and nationwide at least, many senior citizens are choosing to relocate to rural areas for their retirement (Gessert 2004). Rural Texas counties' populations tend to be "grayer" in general than the populations of urban areas, with one-quarter of older adults residing in rural areas (Texas Department on Aging, Office of Aging Policy 2003). Few medical schools provide adequate education in geriatric medicine, and low Medicare reimbursement rates make it difficult to attract young medical students to specialize in geriatric care (Cefalu 2001; see chap. 12).

Many rural counties in Texas are classified as "medically underserved areas/populations" that also qualify as "health professional shortage areas" (Bureau of Health Professions 1995). These rural areas are underserved in that trauma, hospital, and primary care services are limited. The populations are underserved in large part as a result of their composition. Rural Texans are disproportionately low-income, aging, and minority (Hispanic and African American) (Center for Rural Health Initiatives 2001). Health professional shortages include virtually all classes: physicians, nurses, and other allied health professionals. For example, Texas has fewer primary care physicians per 100,000 people than the rest of the United States

(Texas Statewide Health Coordinating Council 2006). Rural Texas has even fewer physicians than the state's metropolitan areas. In fact, in 2005, 23 counties in Texas had no direct patient care physicians at all, and 27 counties lacked any primary care physicians (e.g., family practice, geriatrics, OB/GYN, internal medicine, general pediatrics, and general practice) (Texas Statewide Health Coordinating Council 2006).

Closely connected to health professional shortages are limited emergency medical services and hospital closures. Rural areas often rely on volunteer first responders and EMS providers with only basic emergency medical training (Eskridge 2004). The Texas Department of Health reports that preventable deaths in rural areas could be as much as 85 percent higher than in urban areas (Eskridge 2004). Yet rural areas have an urgent need for emergency medical services. One-third of all motor vehicle accidents nationwide, and two-thirds of the deaths attributed to these accidents, occur on rural roads (Eskridge 2004). In 1999, nearly 60 percent of deaths and 22 percent of injuries due to automobile accidents in Texas occurred in rural Texas (Eskridge 2004).

Between 1990 and 2000, rural Texas led the nation in hospital closures with 24 (Longbotham 2003). As hospitals close their doors, emergency room services are lost and health professionals move away. As a stopgap to help meet the needs of rural Texas residents, rural hospitals and clinics have been established that meet certain criteria to qualify for Medicare reimbursement. Several categories of rural clinics include Critical Access Hospitals (CAH), Rural Health Clinics, and Federally Qualified Health Centers. To receive "critical access hospital" designation, under federal guidelines, a hospital should offer 25 or fewer beds; "[be] located in a rural area; provide 24-hour emergency care services; have an average length of stay of 96 hours or less; and be more than 35 miles from a hospital or another CAH or more than 15 miles in areas with mountainous terrain or only secondary roads OR certified by the State as being a 'necessary provider' of healthcare services to residents in the area" (Centers for Medicare and Medicaid Services 2006; see also chap. 4).

Given that the provision of health care in rural areas can be expensive—with a limited number of providers and professionals, a widely dispersed population, geographical isolation, and economies of scale—the federal government has recognized that a purely private sector solution to the hospital shortage is not practicable. Thus, the federal government created the special class of entities called Rural Health Clinics, which, if small enough, would also qualify for enhanced Medicare and Medicaid reimbursement and could function primarily through the services of midlevel "physician extenders," such as nurse practitioners and physician's assistants. These clinics provide primary health care services. Presently, 381 Rural Health Clinics exist in Texas. Federally Qualified Health Centers are similar to Rural Health Clinics; both exist under the auspices of Medicare and Medicaid (Health Resources and Services Administration 2006). The intent of both is to "help make health care available in communities or to individuals where it might be difficult or impossible using traditional fee-for-service or capitated payment methodologies" (Health Resources and Services Administration 2006).

Medical Problems of Rural Elderly People

Urban and rural persons have similar geriatric syndromes: heart disease, arthritis, incontinence, hip fractures/osteoporosis, and other chronic ailments such as diabetes, emphysema, and head injury. Rural elderly people likewise experience mental health problems such as depression, dementia, delirium, and Alzheimer disease in proportions similar to those of urban elderly people (Vanek 2002). Behavioral issues, sometimes compounded by medical problems, such as substance abuse (especially alcohol and prescription drugs), poor nutrition, and lack of exercise leading to muscle weakness and mobility problems are common in elderly populations. Another pervasive issue is long-term care, whether provided by family caregivers, assisted-living facilities, or nursing homes (see chap. 1). The full panoply of end-of-life issues is particularly relevant to elderly rural populations: advance care planning, palliative care, pain management, and psychological issues of grief and loss.

Mental Health and Rural Elderly People

Another problem for the geriatric population is access to mental health services. Mental health services are scarce in rural areas to begin with (Vanek 2002; see chap. 7). Combined with the general scarcity of geriatric practitioners in rural areas, it is clear that precious few geriatric mental health specialists practice in rural areas, especially outside institutional settings. Further, many elderly patients with mental health problems—such as depression or dementia—are in denial about their need for treatment (Sevush and Leve 1993). Even when family members advise or encourage treatment, the afflicted person is often reluctant to consult a mental health professional. For example, a retired rural laborer who was deeply depressed in part about his chronic pain was finally persuaded by his family to seek psychiatric care for his suicidal ideation. After traveling 100 miles to the nearest psychiatric facility, he was hospitalized. After a week of inpatient treatment—clearly inadequate for his condition—his insurance utilization reviewer declined to certify him for continued hospitalization. His psychiatrist failed to challenge the denial and discharged the patient to his family without providing adequate instructions about his condition or his care. A follow-up outpatient visit was not scheduled for two months. Ten days after the patient returned home, still depressed and suicidal with no supportive services available in his area, he hanged himself. Needless to say, a malpractice lawsuit was filed against the hospital, the psychiatrist, and the utilization review agents. The case was settled out of court for a sizable award to the plaintiff. Even with the premature discharge, the tragedy might have been prevented if local mental health services had been available.

Even though some rural elderly people may be psychologically better off if they remain with family members, in-home care by family creates other problems. When untrained family members become de facto caregivers, they often are confronted with intolerable burdens.[4] Even if family members are willing to assume care-giving responsibilities for relatives with mild dementia or frail elderly relatives, many problems may arise. If the caregivers work and must leave a relative alone for periods of time, falls or other injuries are serious risks. If the family caregiver provides full-time services, burnout and even elder abuse are additional risks (Vitaliano and Katon 2006).

Adjusting to reduced physical and mental capacities may be difficult, especially for persons accustomed to independence and self-sufficiency. One particular problem for rural elderly people is depression, often associated with the disability or death of other relatives. The survivor, who often also becomes a caretaker and caregiver, may suffer from exhaustion and burnout. Colleagues in rural Indiana have reported that family caregivers themselves often decline and deteriorate after a loved one enters a nursing home or dies (personal communication with William J. Winslade). This problem is particularly difficult in rural areas where home health services are in short supply.

Financial considerations often limit private health services, and many rural residents see public programs—even if they are eligible, say, through Medicare for long-term care—as unwanted welfare (Allen 2000; see chap. 10). Family members may also feel guilty about seeking institutionalized care for a relative (Griffith 2004). A former medical student described vividly how her elderly grandmother reluctantly moved to a nursing home because of her physical disability. Her grandmother, who was cognitively intact except for slight memory deficits, was so unhappy in the nursing home that she returned to live with her daughter after a few months. Although it imposed significant burdens on the working caregivers, they acquiesced to the grandmother out of a combination of love and guilt.

In addition to physical isolation, elderly rural Texans who begin to experience chronic problems of aging may also suffer psychological consequences if their fragile health and networks of social support diminish. Loneliness and depression are potentially serious side effects of the loss of mobility and connections with others. Even persons who enjoy being alone feel threatened if their solitude is imposed on them rather than chosen. For rural elderly Texans with significant medical needs and limited family or social support, both access to health care and preservation of autonomy become problematic.

Diminished Autonomy and Independence

The average life expectancy in the United States almost doubled between 1900 and 1965 (Centers for Disease Control and Prevention 2006). Much of the decline in mortality was a result of improved social conditions, such as public health measures, rather than advances in medical care (Centers for Disease Control and Prevention 1999). Until the 1980s it was assumed that even with better medical care that the average life expectancy was about 75 years. However, it is now well-documented that longevity in the United States continues to increase. Average life expectancy for women is now nearly 80 years and 74 years for men, and mortality rates are declining most rapidly for persons who are over 85 (Centers for Disease Control and Prevention 2006). A PBS Frontline special reported that this age group will expand from 5 to 20 million over the next twenty years; it is the "fastest-growing segment of the U.S. population" (2006). The increase in longevity is a result of both preventive health measures and medical advances, with the decline in mortality from cardiovascular

disease being the single-most significant factor. However, as our population lives longer, chronic diseases such as Alzheimer's, dementia, COPD,
kidney failure, hypertension, congestive heart failure, and others typically
accompany greater longevity. Although many older people cope with
chronic disease without significant physical or mental disability, studies
show that as longevity increases, so also does the likelihood of dependency and disability (Cassel, Rudberg, and Olshansky 1992).

Rural elderly persons often highly value their independence and resist
institutional care even if it is available.[5] Although not unique to rural
elderly people, impaired memory, cognitive abilities, hearing, and vision
create problems of mobility and judgment that may be exacerbated for
persons in rural areas. For one thing, elderly persons are more vulnerable
to falls that cause head injuries and broken bones. Older persons experience medical problems that impair their ability to drive, and persons in
rural settings rarely have access to public transportation. In contrast to
urban areas or even rural Indiana where low-cost public transportation is
available, rural Texans depend almost exclusively on cars or trucks. A
rural physician once asked what he should do about an elderly patient of
his who he felt was incompetent to drive because of her poor eyesight and
hearing. He felt that she was a danger to others and herself, but he knew
that if she did not drive she could be stranded in the boondocks. For rural
Texans mobility is a major concern. But the physician's concern about his
patient's judgment is well founded. Drivers over 70, like teenaged drivers,
account for a disproportionately large number of traffic accidents and
fatalities (U.S. Department of Transportation National Highway Traffic
Safety Administration 2000). As noted earlier, rural highways are particularly dangerous. All these factors threaten the autonomy of elderly people,
especially those who live alone or in remote locations such as farms or
ranches. Loss of autonomy for persons who are by nature more independent can also be a severe psychological setback.

Race, Culture, and the Rural Elderly People of Texas

Cultural diversity among elderly rural Texans poses challenges. The
ethnic mix in East Texas, for example, features a high percentage of African
Americans, while in West Texas a significant percentage of the population
is Hispanic (Texas State Data Center and Office of the State Demographer
2007). Robert Weinick and colleagues (2000) established that Hispanic

and African American populations are underserved in terms of health care; they are less likely to be insured and less likely to make use of the health care that is available to them. Compounded with the lack of access in rural areas, rural minorities in Texas represent an especially poorly served population in terms of health care—particularly when members of those minority groups happen to be elderly.

Cultural differences in rural populations affect access to health care services. The rural Caucasian population is more likely to use available health care services than the African American or Hispanic population (Weinick, Zuvekas, and Cohen 2000). Part of the explanation is that the former have higher incomes and higher expectations from and better information about health professionals and services. The elderly African American population in general is less likely to seek primary care services; access is more often sought when trauma or emergency care is needed (Zuvekas and Taliaferro 2003). In turn, the Hispanic population is inclined to rely on family support first and only later turn to health professionals (Talamantes, Lindeman, and Mouton 2007). For example, Hispanic males might be reluctant to seek health care unless their wives encourage and support it (Rich and Ro 2002). With Hispanic rural Texans, another complication is the language barrier.

Rural Texans, especially minorities, may be more likely to use home remedies or alternative medicine before consulting physicians, partly because of costs and other problems of access and partly because of doubts about or distrust toward the health care system (Smith 2001). Even when physicians are consulted for medical problems such as congestive heart failure or depression, rural residents may not abandon alternative remedies, so deep-seated are some of these traditions. The continued use of home remedies by rural elderly persons presents problems if and when they do seek medical treatment. Sometimes alternative remedies—such as gingko biloba, which is taken because it is believed by some to alleviate memory loss—may cause negative drug interactions with pharmaceuticals such as diuretics or antidepressants (Cupp 1999; University of Maryland Medical Center Medical References 2002). Health professionals treating rural geriatric patients need to inquire, and patients need to be educated about drug interactions.

Lacking Insurance

Another dimension of the access to care problem is that a substantial portion of the entire Texas population—approximately 25 percent—lacks health insurance (DeNavas-Walt, Proctor, and Lee 2005). This is the highest percentage of uninsured persons in the United States (DeNavas-Walt, Proctor, and Lee 2005). Although many rural Texans are by virtue of their poverty eligible for Medicaid, many persons are discouraged by bureaucratic obstacles to enrollment, as well as an aversion to the stigma of "welfare" (Gennetian, Redcross, and Miller 2006). Others, such as the low-income rural working poor, are ineligible for Medicaid but unable to afford health insurance. Still others who are indigent are eligible for county health services, but many counties lack resources to provide more than minimal health care services (Hermer and Winslade 2004).

Rural, Elderly, and Incarcerated

A special problem of access to care exists for aging prison populations in Texas. It might seem that prison populations are not "rural" in the same sense as senior citizens who have either chosen a rural life or remain in a rural setting for lack of other options. Nonetheless, most Texas prisons are located in rural areas (Texas Department of Criminal Justice 2007). Some commentators cynically observe that incarcerated elderly people may, in some instances, receive superior care to their noncriminal counterparts (Henson 2007). Regardless of whether this is true, as with the elderly population in general, the population of inmates who are elderly is increasing rapidly. In fact, it is increasing "faster than any other inmate age group," in no small part because inmates tend to age faster because of their lives of risky behavior and poor health care (Criminal Justice Policy Council 1999). The Texas prison population now exceeds 150,000 prisoners, many of whom have long mandatory sentences with little prospect for parole (Legislative Budget Board 2007). Many of these inmates are older repeat offenders with chronic or degenerative diseases (Trevino 2005). As a whole, the prison population has a lower health status and greater medical needs than their free-world counterparts. In addition, a substantial number of Texas inmates have untreated mental disorders and/or impaired cognitive capacities (Ward 2007), which raises ethical and legal issues concerning informed consent to treatment.

In response to the needs of these inmates, the Texas Department of Criminal Justice has established geriatric services as well as palliative and hospice care for elderly and terminally ill inmates (Texas Department of Criminal Justice 2006). As with rural areas, however, the prison health care system has a shortage of mental health professionals as well as geriatric expertise. Even when aging or terminally ill prisoners are granted compassionate parole, however, it follows that, having been incarcerated for so long, many have little, if any, family or community support awaiting them outside the prison walls. As indigent, solitary parolees, they often face more formidable access to health care problems than they did as inmates.

Implications for Ethical Practices

What implications do these dilemmas have for older rural Texans? Education about the needs of geriatric rural patients is imperative. For those who experience chronic illness without significant disability, there will be a greater need for geriatric health care services. Because it is difficult to provide specialized geriatric care for sparsely populated rural areas, primary care health providers need enhanced geriatric education. But education of health professionals alone is not enough. Additional education is needed for family caregivers as well as patients who can and may want to manage their own care.

Rural Texans, unlike many of their urban elderly counterparts, do not have the optional living arrangements of retirement communities, assisted living, senior services, or other group options. If rural elderly Texans in frontier or border counties have physical or mental disabilities that require caretaking beyond what family members can provide, they have few local options other than a nursing home or relocation to a remote facility. For many Texans this option would be unpalatable even if it did exist (Phillips, Hawes, and Leyk Williams 2004). Moreover, many nursing homes in Texas have been under constant criticism for inadequate staffing and services (Minority Staff Special Investigations Division Committee on Government Reform U.S. House of Representatives 2002). In addition, numerous lawsuits for negligence as well as criminal actions have been filed against nursing homes (Diversicare Gen. Partner, Inc. v. Rubio 2005). Also, the Texas legislature is in the process of evaluating and revising regulations pertaining to nursing homes. Quality of care in nursing homes and other long-term care facilities, such as group homes, is a major bioethics issue as well as a governmental concern in Texas. (William J. Winslade is part of a legal-ethical consulting team that is reviewing for the Texas legislature not only nursing home regulation but also a wide range of issues concerning financing, quality of care, and public and private responsibilities for long-term care in Texas.)

Unless the projected shortage of geriatric medical professionals is eased, creative stopgap solutions will be required. One example that could be duplicated in other rural areas of Texas is the East Texas Geriatric Education Center at the University of Texas Medical Branch (UTMB). It is funded by the federal government and was established to train health professionals already in the area to provide better care for geriatric patients. The UTMB Geriatric Education Center offers teleconference seminars on health problems mentioned previously that are common among rural geriatric patients. In addition, education is offered related to medical bioethics issues such as advance care planning, health insurance, palliative care and pain management, end-of-life care, and grief management. The Texas Tech University School of Medicine, based in Lubbock, is expanding all over West Texas; similar education initiatives could be provided through this university. As our elderly population continues to increase, we will need even more geriatric specialists. Rural areas not only lack health professionals but also need health professionals trained specifically to treat geriatric patients.

These problems are not easily solved by individuals acting on their own and relying on private resources. Many elderly persons, even if they have Medicare, often do not have enough income to pay for long-term care services. Reliance on savings is unreliable because it is difficult to predict how much care an individual will need. Private insurance is not available to those who already have long-term care needs, and a substantial number of elderly persons have modest incomes. Although Medicaid is a long-term care safety net for those eligible for it, many elderly persons with incomes too high to qualify for Medicaid have incomes too low to purchase long-term care in the private sector. Commentators like Judith Feder and Sheila Burke (2007) have argued that long-term care for elderly people—as well as persons younger than 65 who need it—is a public responsibility. At the very least it is reasonable and prudent for the government to provide expenses for catastrophic care. Yet when legislation was passed to add catastrophic care to Medicare, AARP launched a successful campaign to repeal the legislation because it increased Medicare premiums. As long-term care needs are increasing, especially for elderly people, perhaps it is time to reconsider what role the public health care system should now play in providing long-term care.

For free-market fundamentalists, who abound in a state as conservative as Texas, it might be tempting to dismiss the health care problems of rural elderly people as a matter of market efficiency. Proportionally, rural elderly people are a small part of the population, and given the many problems involved in providing sufficient access to health care, the costs of ministering to their needs are high. If one accepts that a private-sector solution to the problem of caring for Texas's rural elderly people is unlikely, given the lack of profitability, then it appears necessary for the government to step in. Otherwise, the state faces an ethical dilemma: It will not be caring for a growing, vulnerable segment of its population.

NOTES

1. A "frontier" county is one whose population density is less than seven persons per square mile (Center for Rural Health Initiatives 2001). A "border" county is one along the Texas-Mexico border, usually within 100 miles of the border (Center for Rural Health Initiatives 2001).

2. The Panhandle measures some 25,610 square miles, comprising some 26 counties (Rathjen 2007). The total population of the area, as of the 2000 census, was 402,862. However, this figure does include the more populous cities of Amarillo and Canyon. Panhandle counties are smaller and more densely populated than their far West Texas counterparts. This chapter focuses primarily on rural West Texas because in its geographical isolation, its situation embodies many of the biggest problems faced by rural elderly people.

3. Physician recruitment is a longstanding challenge. For example, in 1993 the *Dallas Morning News* ran an article about the difficulties inherent in drawing doctors to the West Texas desert (Loe 1993). Small rural towns lack the cultural amenities that many newly minted physicians may desire nor can they usually offer salaries as high as those paid in urban areas (Loe 1993). To better illustrate the shortage of health care professionals in rural West Texas, it should be noted that as of February 2001, Presidio and Terrell Counties had no primary care physicians (Texas Department of Health Center for Health Statistics 2004).

4. In Hispanic families, family members are often the de facto caregivers. As in

other cultures, children are expected to take in their elders, and it can be shameful if they do not. There is a strong cultural preference in the Hispanic community for elders to live with their children (Talamantes, Lindeman, and Mouton 2007).

5. The stereotype of rural seniors is that they are highly independent. Yet it can be difficult to determine whether or not rural elderly people, in Texas or elsewhere, are truly fiercely independent or just dealing with the reality that there are simply fewer nursing homes available to them than to their urban counterparts (Bane 1996).

REFERENCES

Allen, B. E. 2000. The price of reform: Cost-sharing proposals for the Medicare home health benefit. *Yale Journal on Regulation* 17 (1): 137–94.
American Geriatric Society, Core Writing Group of the Task Force on the Future of Geriatric Medicine. 2005. Caring for older Americans: The future of geriatric medicine. *Journal of the American Geriatric Society* 53:S245–56.
Associated Press. 2004. Van Horn hospital closing due to finances. *Midland Reporter-Telegram.* www.mywesttexas.com/site/news.cfm?newsid=11885370& BRD=2288&PAG=461&dept_id=475626&rfi=8 (accessed April 2, 2007).
Bane, S. D. 1996. *Mental health and aging training for service providers.* Kansas City: National Resource Center for Rural Elderly, University of Missouri–Kansas City.
Bureau of Health Professions. 1995. *Guidelines for medically underserved area and population designations.* U.S. Department of Health and Human Services. http://bhpr.hrsa.gov/shortage/muaguide.htm (accessed August 12, 2004).
Cassel, C. K., M. A. Rudberg, and S. J. Olshansky. 1992. The price of success: Health care in an aging society. *Health Affairs (Millwood)* 11 (2): 87–99.
Cefalu, C. A. 2001. Patients in Peril: Critical Shortages in Geriatric Care. Testimony presented before the Special Committee on Aging, United States Senate, February 27, 2002, on behalf of the American Geriatrics Society / Louisiana Geriatrics Society. American Geriatrics Society. www.americangeriatrics.org/news/aging breauxtestimony.shtml (accessed February 29, 2008).
Center for Rural Health Initiatives. 2001. *Rural health in Texas 1999–2000: A report to the governor and the 77th legislature.* Austin: Texas Department of Health.
Centers for Disease Control and Prevention. 1999. Ten great public health achievements, United States, 1900–1999. *Morbidity and Mortality Weekly Report* 48 (12): 241–43.
———. 2006. *Health, United States, 2006, with chartbook on trends in the health of Americans.* U.S. Department of Health and Human Services, Centers for Disease Control and Prevention, National Center for Health Statistics. www.cdc .gov/nchs/data/hus/hus06.pdf# (accessed March 29, 2007).

Centers for Medicare and Medicaid Services. 2006. *Critical Access Hospital program.* U.S. Department of Health and Human Services. www.cms.hhs.gov/ MLNProducts/downloads/2006cah.pdf (accessed April 1, 2007).

Criminal Justice Policy Council. 1999. *Elderly offenders in Texas prisons.* Texas Department of Criminal Justice. www.lbb.state.tx.us/PubSafety_CrimJustice/6_ Links/ElderlyOffenders.pdf (accessed April 2, 2007).

Cupp, M. J. 1999. Herbal remedies: Adverse effects and drug interactions. *American Family Physician* 59 (5): 1239. www.aafp.org/afp/990301ap/1239.html (accessed April 5, 2007).

DeNavas-Walt, C., B. D. Proctor, and C. H. Lee. 2005. *Income, poverty, and health insurance coverage in the United States, 2004.* Current Population Reports: Consumer Income. U.S. Census Bureau. www.census.gov/prod/2005pubs/ p60–229.pdf (accessed April 5, 2007).

Diversicare Gen. Partner, Inc. v. Rubio. 2005. In *185 S.W.3d 842:* Tex. 2005.

Eskridge, C. 2004. *Trauma stabilization services in rural Texas.* Texas Legislative Council. www.tlc.state.tx.us/pubspol/traumaservrural.pdf (accessed April 2, 2007).

Feder, J., and S. Burke. 2007. *A message from Judith Feder and Sheila Burke, policy perspective: What about long-term care?* Georgetown University Long-Term Care Financing Project. http://ltc.georgetown.edu/federburke.html (accessed April 2, 2007).

Frontline. 2006. Introduction to "Living Old." Public Broadcast System. www.pbs .org/wgbh/pages/frontline/livingold/etc/synopsis.html (accessed March 28, 2007).

Gennetian, L. A., C. Redcross, and C. Miller. 2006. Policy and practitioner perspective: Regional differences in the effects of welfare reform: Evidence from an experimental program in rural and urban Minnesota. *Georgetown Journal of Poverty Law and Policy* 119: 1–27.

Gessert, C. 2004. Rural/urban differences in end-of-life care: Reflections on social contracts. In *Nevada Center for Ethics and Health Policy 2004 Symposium on Rural Bioethics.* Reno, NV.

Griffith, V. 2004. Generations to come: Researcher examines options for Latino elders as economic realities challenge family traditions. University of Texas Austin Feature Story. www.utexas.edu/features/archive/2004/latino.html (accessed March 29, 2007).

Health Resources and Services Administration. 2006. *Comparison of the rural health clinic and federally qualified health center programs.* U.S. Department of Health and Human Services. www.ask.hrsa.gov/downloads/fqhc-rhccomparison .pdf (accessed April 1, 2007).

Henson, S. 2005. Elderly inmates health costs rising. http://gritsforbreakfast.blogspot .com. (accessed April 2, 2007).

Hermer, L. D., and W. J. Winslade. 2004. Access to health care in Texas: A patient-centered perspective. *Texas Tech Law Review* 35 (1): 33–99.

Legislative Budget Board. 2007. *Current correctional population indicators: Adult and juvenile correctional populations monthly report.* Texas Legislative Budget Board. www.lbb.state.tx.us/PubSafety_CrimJustice/2_Current_Corr_Pop_Indicators/MonthlyReport.pdf. (accessed April 5, 2007).

Loe, V. 1993. A crisis in isolation: Despite lavish offers, rural areas have difficulty attracting doctors. *Dallas Morning News,* Nov. 28.

Longbotham, R. L. 2003. A rural Texan talks about policy and health care in rural Texas. *Texas Journal of Rural Health* 21 (3): 39, 41.

Minority Staff Special Investigations Division Committee on Government Reform U.S. House of Representatives. 2002. *Nursing home conditions in Texas: Many nursing homes fail to meet federal standards for adequate care.* U.S. House of Representatives. http://oversight.house.gov/Documents/20040830114327–83314.pdf (accessed April 2, 2007).

Moynihan, D. P. 1996. *Columbia world of quotations.* www.bartleby.com (accessed April 2, 2007).

Murdock, S. H., T. Swenton, N. Hoque, B. Pecotte, and S. White. 2000. *Demographic and socioeconomic change in rural Texas: Report prepared for the House Select Committee on Rural Development.* College Station, TX: Center for Demographic and Socioeconomic Research and Education, Department of Rural Sociology, Texas A&M University.

Ozeki, R. 1998. *My year of meats.* New York: Viking Penguin.

Phillips, C. D., C. Hawes, and M. Leyk Williams. 2004. Nursing homes in rural and urban areas, 2001. Texas A&M University System Health Science Center, School of Rural Public Health, Southwest Rural Health Research Center. www.srph.tamhsc.edu/centers/srhrc/NHRUA01.htm (accessed April 2, 2007).

Rathjen, F. W. 2007. Panhandle. University of Texas at Austin. www.tsha.utexas.edu/handbook/online/articles/PP/ryp1.html (accessed April 5, 2007).

Rich, J. A., and M. Ro. 2002. A poor man's plight: Uncovering the disparity in men's health. Community Voices. W. K. Kellogg Foundation 2007. www.community voices.org/Uploads/coo2vwbbgpaulnjtmq2ksu55_20020826104857.pdf. (accessed April 2, 2007).

Sevush, S., and N. Leve. 1993. Denial of memory deficit in Alzheimer's disease. *American Journal of Psychiatry* 150 (5): 748–51.

Smith, G. L. 2001. An ethnographic study of home remedy use for African-American children. Ph.D. diss., School of Nursing, University of Texas School of Health Sciences at Houston, Houston, TX.

Talamantes, M., R. Lindeman, and C. Mouton. 2007. Health and health care of Hispanic/Latino American elders. Ethnogeriatric Curriculum Module. www.stanford.edu/group/ethnoger/hispaniclatino.html#V. (accessed March 29, 2007).

Texas Department of Criminal Justice. 2006. ESTELLE (E2) CID—Prison. www.tdcj.state.tx.us/stat/unitdirectory/e2.htm (accessed April 5, 2007).

———. 2007. Unit directory-region/type of facility/map. www.tdcj.state.tx.us/stat/unitdirectory/map.htm (accessed April 5, 2007).

Texas Department of Health, Center for Health Statistics. 2004. 2005–2010 Texas

State Health Plan. Austin: Texas Statewide Health Coordinating Council, Texas Dept. of State Health Services.

Texas Department on Aging, Office of Aging Policy. 2003. Texas demographics: Older adults in Texas. www.dads.state.tx.us/news_info/publications/studies/NewDemoProfileHi-Rez-4-03.pdf. (accessed April 2, 2007).

Texas State Data Center and Office of the State Demographer. 2007. Texas redistricting plan—P. L. 94–171. Business and Industry Data Center Meeting, April 19–20 2007. http://txsdc.utsa.edu/data/census/2000/redistrict/pl94–171/desctab/re_tab4.txt (accessed April 5, 2007).

Texas Statewide Health Coordinating Council. 2006. Chapter 2: Status of the health workforce in Texas. Department of State Health Services. www.dshs.state.tx.us/chs/shcc/reports/PCChap2%20072406.pdf. (accessed April 5, 2007).

Trevino, R. 2005. High cost of seniors serving time in Texas prisons. KHOU. www.khou.com/news/local/stories/khou051214_gj_elderlyinmates.df1c82f.html. (accessed April 2, 2007).

University of Maryland Medical Center Medical References. 2002. Gingko biloba. Complementary and Alternative Medicine Index. www.umm.edu/altmed/ConsHerbs/GinkgoBilobach.html (accessed April 5, 2007).

U.S. Census Bureau. 2007. Texas quick facts. http://quickfacts.census.gov/qfd/states/48000.html (accessed April 2, 2007).

U.S. Department of Transportation National Highway Traffic Safety Administration. 2000. Traffic safety facts 2000. www.nrd.nhtsa.dot.gov/pdf/nrd-30/ncsa/tsf2000/2000oldpop.pdf. (accessed April 5, 2007).

Valdez, D. W. 2004. Van Horn hospital to close. *El Paso Times,* June 5.

Vanek, D. 2002. Ruralfacts: Rural mental health. Research and Training Center on Disability in Rural Communities. http://rtc.ruralinstitute.umt.edu/MentalHealth.htm. (accessed March 29, 2007).

Vitaliano, P. P., and W. J. Katon. 2006. Effects of stress on family caregivers: Recognition and management. *Psychiatric Times* 23 (7): 23.

Ward, M. 2007. Texas selected for study of mental health illnesses in state prisons: Nearly a third of state, county jail inmates have mental health diseases. *Austin American-Statesman*, Feb. 19, 2007. www.statesman.com/news/content/region/legislature/stories/02/20/20mental.html. (accessed April 12, 2007).

Weinick, R. M., S. H. Zuvekas, and J. W. Cohen. 2000. Racial and ethnic differences in access to and use of health care services, 1977 to 1996. *Medical Care Research and Review* 57 Suppl 1: 36–54.

Zuvekas, S. H., and G. S. Taliaferro. 2003. Pathways to access: Health insurance, the health care delivery system, and racial/ethnic disparities, 1996–1999. *Health Affairs (Millwood)* 22 (2): 139–53.

CHAPTER 12

Supporting the Rural Physician

Processes and Programs

JAMIE ANDERSON, M.S., M.A., AND
CRAIG M. KLUGMAN, PH.D

This strange town, primitive and isolated, entombed by the
mountains, with no places of amusement, not even a cinema,
nothing but its grim mine, its quarries and ore works, its string of
chapels and bleak rows of houses—a queer and silently contained community.

Cronin 1937, p. 32

This central room was at once business office, consultation room,
operating-theater, living-room, poker den, and warehouse for
guns and fishing tackle. Against a brown plaster wall was a
cabinet of zoological collections and medical curiosities.

Lewis 1925, p. 7

The doctor was the entire staff.

Hertzler 1938, p. 129

The challenge of providing medical care to rural and frontier
regions has long been difficult. In Archibald Joseph Cronin's novel *The
Citadel* (1937), the fictional Dr. Andrew Manson becomes sole provider to
a Welsh mining town. For Sinclair Lewis in the 1920s, being a rural physician meant working in the backwaters of medical practice. It also often
meant a lack of resources (Geyman, Norris, and Hart 2001). Arthur Hertzler (1938) discusses in his memoir the essence of the lack of support that
many rural physicians felt and still feel (see part 2). Rural health care providers must be generalists (Geyman, Norris, and Hart 2001; see chap. 8).

While the physicians described by Cronin and Lewis are fictional, Hertzler reminds us that for a long time there has been recognition that in reality providing quality medical care to a small population living over a large geographic expanse requires creative solutions. Simply importing the urban model of a concentrated hospital or medical center does not work. In Australia, part of the solution has been the flying doctor's service. In China, there has been a tradition of the barefoot doctor, walking from town to town to provide care in rural areas. And in the United States, the tradition of the frontier doctor meant that the physician had to practice mostly alone to provide all possible health care services to his or her patients, as portrayed in the fictional television show *Doctor Quinn, Medicine Woman*. In this chapter, we briefly review the particular demographic challenges facing the rural practitioner and then investigate potential solutions: community-based medical education (CBME) and community-based participatory research (CBPR). CBME is when medical students learn by participating in community medical practice, such as clinics, community hospitals, and private offices, where practicing, nonacademic physicians teach them. In CBPR medical experts work in equal partnership with community members and groups to pursue research that will improve the health of the members of the society. CBME and CBPR programs geared toward undergraduate, graduate, and professional medical education work to increase the number of physicians who practice and who want to practice in rural areas.

The Rural Landscape

Rurality has much to do with scarcity—the scarcity of resources (people, money, technical support) and scarcity of alternatives or options. The truth about life in rural and remote areas is that there are numerous truths (Turner 2005). Rural areas have more primary care Health Professions Shortage Areas, a higher percentage of poverty, more patients with chronic disease, a greater percentage of elderly persons, and a greater proportion of patients receiving Medicare, Medicaid, or without health insurance than nonrural areas (Rabinowitz et al. 1999). In rural areas, access to care is more limited, populations are sicker, physician and hospital reimbursements are lower, and barriers to retention of the health workforce are greater (Pacheco et al. 2005). The ability to attract and retain physicians is economically critical to these communities, allowing them to keep their hospitals open, create health-related jobs, and thereby attract businesses and retirees to settle there (Pacheco et al. 2005).

Understanding the factors that contribute to the recruitment and retention of physicians in rural areas is crucial if the populations in these areas are to be effectively served (see chaps. 6 and 7). From 1990 to 2000, the overall number of physicians practicing in rural areas increased, but the proportion relative to urban areas continued to decline (Brooks et al. 2002). Simply recruiting new physicians is therefore unlikely to improve the longstanding shortage of rural physicians unless long-term retention is also increased (Rabinowitz et al. 2005). Rural practitioners are often more involved in higher-level assessment emergency care due to the high incidence of trauma in rural areas, procedural-based work, obstetrics, anesthetics, surgery, and community-based care than their urban counterparts (Ypinazar and Margolis 2006). Rural health care delivery systems are smaller and less well staffed than their urban counterparts: 20 percent of the U.S. population lives in rural areas, but only 9 percent of physicians practice in those areas (Rosenblatt et al. 2006). Rural Community Health Centers report significantly higher proportions of unfilled positions and more difficulty recruiting family physicians than their urban counterparts, and more than one-third of rural grantees have been recruiting for a family physician for seven or more months (Rosenblatt et al. 2006). The lack of spousal employment opportunities, lack of cultural activities and opportunities, lack of adequate housing, and poor-quality schools were perceived as disproportionately greater barriers for rural centers trying to recruit (Rosenblatt et al. 2006).

Community-based medical education is a supporting factor in both recruitment and retention of rural physicians and has received particular attention around the world (Rourke and Frank 2005; Tolhurst, Adams, and Stewart 2006). When urban-background students are exposed to rural practice and a range of rural locations, many of them become interested in rural practice. This exposure may increase the number of students who decide to enter rural practice (Tolhurst, Adams, and Stewart 2006). From an international perspective, studies suggest that empathy and sympathy for the less fortunate may be qualities lacking in doctors who are not exposed to rural life (Giri and Shankar 2006).

U.S. medical schools have been slow to recognize contributions made by community-based faculty (Baldor et al. 2001). However, these schools are becoming increasingly reliant on community-based doctors for ambulatory clinical teaching, especially in the primary care specialties (Bardella et al. 2005). As a result, there has been a large-scale move toward increasing community-based medical education within the medical schools' curriculum with students assigned to a community-based general/family practice physician. When the community is in a rural area, this approach has been a positive influence on selection of rural practice as a career choice (Margolis, Davies, and Ypinazar 2005). There are also positive benefits to established rural practitioners, with enhanced job satisfaction and consequently a positive impact on rural retention (Margolis, Davies, and Ypinazar 2005; Worley et al. 2000). Early experience increased recruitment to primary care / rural medical practice in the United States. These experiences helped students build positive attitudes toward primary care / rural practice (Dornan et al. 2006). Such efforts through the medical school can provide rural medical students and physicians with many benefits though curriculum development, research support, and professional development, ideas that are explored in the next section.

The Role of the Medical School in Rural Health Care

Nationally and in almost every state, policy makers and educators continue to face the challenge of finding effective ways to increase the supply of rural physicians. For the past few decades, a small number of medical schools have developed programs designed to address this problem (Rabinowitz et al. 1999). Successful community-based medical education programs strongly suggest that medical schools have the ability to make a substantial and long-term impact on the rural physician workforce (Rabinowitz et al. 2005). Student and resident rotations have been cited as an important factor in physician recruitment (Brown and Birnbaum 2005). Community-based preceptors teach because they enjoy teaching and the opportunity to stay current (Bowen and Irby 2002). General practitioners who teach report increased morale and job satisfaction (DeWitt 2006).

Networks and relationships are essential to help alleviate the possible isolation well recognized in rural medical life (Baker, Eley, and Lasserre 2005). The keystone to programs that aim to increase rural physician recruitment and development is the community-focused medical school. This relationship with a medical school often begins with a clinical faculty appointment—the official recognition of the academic affiliation. This academic appointment has been perceived to be a distinct benefit

(Baldor et al. 2001; Smyth 2003; Smucny et al. 2005). It helps to reduce professional isolation and results in professional pride about one's role as a preceptor (Walters et al. 2005). In most medical schools, there are limited benefits that accompany a clinical faculty appointment. At the University of Nevada School of Medicine (UNSOM), for example, benefits for rural-based clinical faculty include student contact, the unique opportunity to contribute to an important and influential experience in a student's medical education; a UNSOM Certificate, a formal acknowledgment that can be displayed in the office; waiting room cards, which inform patients that their physician has been selected to participate in the UNSOM Office-Based Clinical Teaching Program; educational workshops—preceptors receive a fee waiver for all continuing medical education activities offered through UNSOM; a staff identification card; library privileges for access to electronic journals, textbooks, and databases, as well as consultation with library staff on information resources; and grant-in-aid waivers, which entitle the preceptor to enroll in university courses systemwide at no tuition cost.

Preceptor benefits are a part of the infrastructure that is an essential element in the success of community-based medical education. This infrastructure has multiple dimensions. Schools of medicine often have Area Health Education Centers (AHECs). The mission of AHECs is to improve the supply, distribution, diversity, and quality of the health workforce, ultimately increasing access to health care in medically underserved areas (see chap. 11). AHECs link the resources of the university health science center with local planning, educational, and clinical resources. This network of health-related institutions provides multidisciplinary educational services to students, faculty, and local practitioners, ultimately improving health care delivery in medically underserved areas. The AHEC program is a long-term initiative, requiring major changes in the traditional method of training medical and other health professions students and in the relationship between university health science centers and community health service delivery systems (U.S. Department of Health and Human Resources Bureau of Health Professionals 2006).

Monetary payment, whether as a modest honorarium or as a compensation of lost time/income, is an important benefit within some subsets of community-based preceptors (Baldor et al. 2001; Carney et al. 2005; Levy and Merchant 2005). In a survey of a sampling of primary care physicians in the six-state New England region of the United States, physicians in

Academic Health Centers (AHC) were significantly more likely to rank payment as "very important" to "necessary" than non-AHC physicians. Other physicians gave a higher level of importance to having a faculty appointment and computer linkages for library, clinical information, or e-mail. Appropriate benefit packages must be designed, and, given the variation of what is valued by preceptors, it may be best to individualize benefits rather than use a "one size fits all" approach (Baldor et al. 2001). The goal is to identify the resources that will provide long-term support of community-based faculty. Physician preceptors need support, training, and space to educate students, and schools of medicine cannot continue to rely on preceptors' altruism alone to support medical education (Thistlethwaite 2006).

Schools of medicine have recognized the need for improved *faculty development* for community preceptors and have developed workshops devoted to building precepting skills (Baker, Dalton, and Walker 2003; Bardella et al. 2005; Wilkes et al. 2006). One way that physicians learn how to be good teachers is by experimenting with new methods and reflecting on their results (Wilkes et al. 2006). One example is the One Minute Preceptor (OMP), which involves teaching faculty participants five microskills to improve their abilities in diagnosing learners' knowledge and understanding clinical cases, as well as directing the faculty to provide feedback, correct mistakes, and teach general rules based on their assessments of learners (Eckstrom, Homer, and Bowen 2006). The model has been seen as an effective method of managing patient care and a more effective and efficient way of teaching in the ambulatory care setting (Aagaard, Teherani, and Irby 2004; Irby 1994). Switching the focus from "teaching" to "encouraging learning" improves the experience for the teacher and the student. UNSOM has taught the OMP in statewide and rural-based faculty development workshops with a favorable response from rural preceptors.

Schools of medicine that have a rural focus often collaborate with the federally funded Student/Resident Experiences and Rotations in Community Health (SEARCH) program. The SEARCH program provides health professions students and residents with opportunities to work in interdisciplinary health care teams, thus extending a unique, hands-on, primary care training experience working with people in underserved rural and urban areas. Rural communities that partner with schools of medicine and the SEARCH program for community-based medical education programs gain access to academic resources, the opportunity to network with state and regional organizations, assistance to develop and perform health promotion and disease prevention activities, recruitment of future health care clinicians, and preceptorship opportunities for medical staff (National Health Service Corps 2006).

Curriculum is an important variable that is within the control of the medical school and reflects its commitment to primary care and rural health care (Brooks et al. 2002). Medical school characteristics such as family medicine clerkships, communication skills courses, and curricula in medical ethics, humanities, and social sciences in medicine play a central role in the development of physicians committed to the well-being of others (Pugno et al. 2005). There may be economies of scale to be considered because there is a substantial amount of infrastructure support that is required for this kind of curriculum (Margolis, Davies, and Ypinazar 2005). However, there are also enhanced opportunities for school of medicine outreach that come as a result of a commitment to this type of curriculum.

Research is another potential area of collaboration between schools of medicine and rural communities. The primary underlying objective of medical research must be to further the health and well-being of individuals; the focus of doctor training must be the diffusion of knowledge to assist colleagues in achieving optimum wellness for each patient. As medical schools continue to modify their teaching in response to credible research that uncovers and exposes advances as well as flaws in health care and medical science, the medical community should encourage scientific curiosity, pursue a vigilant stance of scientific integrity, and guard against the appearance of arrogance (Genuis 2006).

Family medicine researchers often engage in research that involves descriptive or epidemiological investigations of various populations, including practice-based networks or entire communities (Hueston et al. 2006). CBPR is a model that would work well for schools of health (medicine, public health, nursing, and allied health science) and rural communities that are engaged in CBME partnerships. CBPR is defined as a collaborative partnership approach to research that involves researchers and community members in all stages of the research process. All partners are considered expert, and each brings knowledge and resources from different experiences. The goals of CBPR are to increase the relevance of research to a community's capacity building and apply the results appropriately to improve health. CBPR is guided by the principle of shared decision making, power, and resources among the participants (Hueston et al. 2006).

Rural physicians often have research ideas but may lack the skills or assistance to perform the research. The unique Rural Summer Studentship Programs (RSSP) at the University of Western Ontario places students with preceptors in small and midsized communities throughout southwestern Ontario where they have an opportunity to perform rural health research, combined with clinical learning, for eight weeks in the summer after the first or second year of medical school. Research support in the early design phase of projects and the ethics review board process is vital because most of the students and rural preceptors have little experience in this regard. The effectiveness of the program has been reflected in the students' positive perceptions of their learning experiences, including knowledge of rural medicine and patient care, as well as project-specific knowledge. Students have also reported the program stimulates their interest in rural medicine. The opportunity for students to be involved in RSSP projects with rural specialists, as well as rural family doctors, gives students a broader choice of experience and potential career influence (Zorzi et al. 2005). In New Mexico, graduates of their rural-based residencies have formed the backbone of a growing primary care practice-based research network, Research Involving Outpatient Settings Network, which has generated more than $4 million in federal research grant funding back to the medical school (Pacheco et al. 2005).

Another example of infrastructure support that schools of medicine are able to offer to their community-based preceptors is the integration of *technology* into their practices. Personal Digital Assistants (PDAs) have been offered as an incentive to preceptors who participate in community-based medical student education. PDAs offer several advantages over textbooks and desktop computers. They can store large amounts of information of specific interest to the practicing physician as well as general resources such as drug and medical information databases and medical calculators, all in a portable, lightweight platform. The University of British Columbia offered its rural family physician preceptors a PDA with preloaded software as an alternative to receiving $450 in remuneration for teaching. Sixty-three percent of rural community preceptors chose to receive the PDA. After one year, 10 percent of those who chose the PDA had not yet used it, and another 44 percent had had difficulty in getting started using their PDA. Despite these technical difficulties, rural family physicians appeared to find PDAs an acceptable reward for teaching, based on the reported use and utility of the PDA. Recipients reported using their PDAs primarily in the clinical setting, with the feeling that the tool had a positive effect on their patient care (Baumgart 2005; Carroll and Christakis 2004; Fischer et al. 2003; Garritty and El Emam 2006; Scott, Wilson, and Gowans 2005).

Schools of medicine can also offer *continuing medical education* (CME) either on site or online to their community-based faculty. There is a critical need for ongoing CME in trauma care and other ongoing skills training relevant to the specificities of rural practice. Appropriately designed, evidence-based online CME can produce objectively measured changes in behavior as well as sustained gains in knowledge that are comparable or superior to those realized from effective live activities (Fordis et al. 2005). A recent study reported that an interactive online CME program produced changes in knowledge and performance in lipid screening and treatment that were comparable or superior to those produced by a live interactive workshop (Fordis et al. 2005). Additionally, there is evidence that online, case-based, intimate partner (domestic) violence CME programs—a topic that is pertinent in rural communities, as discussed in Thomas's chapter in this volume—can improve short-term educational outcomes as effectively as multiple-day live workshops (Short, Surprenant, and Harris 2006).

The proof that such ideas and approaches can work comes from programs that have already tried and often succeeded in improving rural health care. Medical school efforts in Australia, Canada, and the United States seek to improve rural health care provider recruitment, retention, and job satisfaction. Most of these interventions have a strong evaluative component, thus demonstrating their efficacy. The following sections of this chapter discuss exemplary models of rural medical outreach and health care professional development in undergraduate and graduate medical education as well as interprofessional education. This discussion is not exhaustive but represents examples of best practices.

Undergraduate Medical Education

Undergraduate medical students vary considerably in their ability, prior knowledge and experience, interests, career inclination, learning styles, and optimum pace of learning (Leung 2001). Students' attitudes

TABLE 12.1

Exemplary programs in community-based medical education (CBME), graduate medical education (GME), interdisciplinary health education (IHE), and community-based participatory research (CBPR)

Institution/Country	Program Type	Rural Placement	Student Year	Elective/Mandatory
East Tennessee State University (ETSU) *United States*	CBME	Four-week summer elective in Appalachia	All	Elective and offered to non-ETSU students
Flinders University *Australia*	CBME	Full-year rural clinical rotation	Senior students	Elective
James Cook University School of Medicine *Australia*	GME	Rural internship	Final year	Elective
Jefferson Medical College *United States*	CBME	PSAP (third-year clerkship)	All	By invitation / rural track selection required on admission
New South Wales (NSW) Department of Health *Australia*	GME	NSW Rural Resident Medical Officer Cadetship Program	Residents	Mandatory if in program
Ontario *Canada*	GME	Community practice/family residency	Residents	Mandatory if in program
School of Medicine at the University of Queensland *Australia*	GME	Rural clinical internship	Residents	Mandatory if in program
School of Medicine at the University of Queensland *Australia*	CBME	Rural clinical placements	Third	Elective
School of Rural Health University of Melbourne *Australia*	IHE	Rural Interprofessional Education Project sends interdisciplinary teams of students on two-week rural placements	Medicine, health promotion, nursing, pharmacy, physiotherapy, public health	Elective
SUNY Upstate *United States*	CBME	36-week clinical RMED experience	Third	Elective
The Center for Rochester's (NY) Health *United States*	IHE	Interdisciplinary teams of students working with community agencies	Health professional students	Elective

Institution / Country	Type	Program	Level	Status
University of Adelaide *Australia*	CBME	One-week rural program	First and second	Elective
University of Calgary *Canada*	CBME	Four-week rural rotation	Third	Mandatory
University of Iowa *United States*	CBME	Family medicine clerkship	Third	Elective
University of Minnesota Medical School *United States*	CBME	RPAP-36 week	Third	Elective
University of Nebraska Medical Center *United States*	CBME	Family medicine preceptorship	Third	Elective
University of New Mexico School of Medicine *United States*	GME CBPR	Family medicine residency Residents/students	Residents Variable	Mandatory if in program Elective
University of North Dakota School of Medicine and Health Sciences *United States*	CBME, CBPR	Seven months: surgery, family medicine clerkship; partial clerkship: internal medicine, pediatrics, OB/GYN	Third	Elective
University of Tasmania *Australia*	IHE	Rural placement, curriculum, rural health club	Medical, nursing, pharmacy	Elective
University of Western Australia *Australia*	CBME, CBPR	Multiple clinical sites for one year	Fifth	Elective
University of Western Australia *Australia*	CBME	Four-day rural experience	Fourth	Elective
University of Western Ontario Schulich School of Medicine *Canada*	GME CBPR	MSCTN-specialty residency experiences in rural settings Medical students	Residents Second	Mandatory if in program Elective
West Virginia Rural Health Education Partnerships *United States*	IHE	Three-month rural experience	All health professional students	Mandatory

toward particular medical specialties change following their experience in individual clerkships (Ellsbury et al. 1998). Exposing students to rural medicine during the first two years of their undergraduate study has been shown to increase the chance of their choosing rural practice as a career (Wilkinson et al. 2004).

Community-based participatory educational experiences support the students' cognitive processes by seeing diseases in life, rather than in texts, providing a context for their learning, importing a framework to understand clinical practice, showing them the clinician's perspective, and helping them develop clinical ways of thinking. Students learn about the roles and responsibilities of health professionals and the importance of good communication and collaboration, as well as patients' experiences of health and disease and the impact of illness on them (Dornan et al. 2006).

Community-based medical education experiences are usually structured on a one-to-one student/physician basis and are referred to as *preceptorships.* Both men and women become more confident in areas where they were least confident before the preceptorship (Lacy, Paulman, and Hartman 2005). The culture of an ambulatory teaching site is reflected in the attitudes of clinic staff toward learners, the ability of the learners to participate meaningfully in the clinic, and the importance placed on teaching and learning—all of which individually and collectively influence learning. Sites conducive to learning have such characteristics as the opportunity for learners to evaluate patients and acquire clinical skills, a sufficient number of available and effective teachers, sufficient number and variety of patients, an orientation, and sufficient time for teaching (Bowen and Irby 2002).

A "pipeline" approach has been proposed to increase the supply of physicians to rural communities (Geyman et al. 2000; Smucny et al. 2005). This "pipeline" metaphor has been used by Thomas E. Norris to describe a sequence of rurally oriented programs, coordinated through medical schools to nurture and mentor students with an interest in rural health to become rural doctors, based on educational content and experience of rural health (Dunbabin, McEwin, and Cameron 2006; Norris 2005). A key component of this pipeline is providing medical students clinical experiences in rural settings (Smucny et al. 2005). We discuss two of the programs that have put the pipeline concept into practice.

Data from the University of Newcastle, Australia, reported that the students' level of interest in rural practice depends on interaction between students and location factors and other external influences, with students seeking to match their needs and interests with locations. Some are predisposed to develop interest in rural practice because of their familiarity with rural areas, level of altruism, interest in generalist work, and interest in certain leisure activities (Tolhurst, Adams, and Stewart 2006).

The challenge of transferring undergraduate medical training to a rural environment requires a new educational mind-set, an adaptive curriculum, and the resources to implement it (Maley et al. 2006). The shift away from reliance on traditional, highly resourced, typically urban, tertiary-level teaching hospitals has sparked concerns about the lack of teachers and infrastructure to support significant numbers of medical students in rural areas for significant periods (Waters et al. 2006). Much of the research on the University of Washington's regional WWAMI (Washington, Wyoming, Alaska, Montana, and Idaho) program, a rural-based undergraduate medical education curriculum, was aimed at determining if there were differences in university versus community settings. Researchers found overwhelming evidence that students learned just as well in either setting (Irby and Wilkerson 2003).

Exemplary Rural CBME Programs for Medical Students

The challenges of providing rural community-based medical education have been dealt with successfully outside the United States as well. For example, all medical schools in Canada and Australia provide rural training opportunities (Woloschuk and Tarrant 2002). Such programs have a strong impact on student's professional development, increase opportunities for patient contact and hands-on learning, increase rural physician recruitment and retention, increase involvement of rural physicians, and benefit rural communities in improved health and economics.

1. The Parallel Rural Community Curriculum (PRCC) was developed by Flinders University, Australia, in 1997 to enable senior medical students to undertake an entire clinical year based in rural general practice in the Riverland region of South Australia. The aim is to allow students to work with a patient-centered focus, in which they follow patients through the continuum of health services from presentation in primary care to hospital inpatient care and return to the community. In each practice, the physicians' initial worries included concerns about time, clinical exposure, the

organization of the program, and the infrastructure needs of their practices to support students. Partnership development with local stakeholders was the key to successful development of this CBME program (Walters, Worley, and Mugford 2003). Students in this program reported a pattern of increased clinical exposure to common clinical conditions and procedures in comparison with their hospital-based peers. They also reported greater competence in procedures (Worley, Strasser, and Prideaux 2004). PRCC students had five hours and 32 minutes more patient contact time per week than the nonrural students. All students were also offered exactly the same lectures (three to four hours per week), delivered on site at the tertiary hospital and distributed via video-conferencing or videotape to the PRCC students. Despite the predictable difficulties associated with transmission failures, poor picture quality, and lack of interactivity, the remote students actually participated more in this lecture activity than their tertiary hospital colleagues (Worley et al. 2006). The "participatory" learning environment in the PRCC led to a sense of the students feeling valued by staff at the local hospital. This contrasted with the students' descriptions of staff seeming inconvenienced by the students at the tertiary hospital. The PRCC findings should give students confidence that they do not have to sacrifice academic performance when taking advantage of such learning opportunities (Worley, Esterman, and Prideaux 2004).

2. The University of Western Australia (UWA) Rural Clinical School (RCS) is unique among Australian rural clinical schools in that it places small cohorts of fifth-year medical students in multiple remote sites for the full academic year. A small administrative office was set up at each rural site with the purpose of supporting the medical coordinator and students. The medical coordinator (part-time) for each site was an experienced rural and remote practitioner either in private practice locally or on the staff of the regional hospital. Most of the academic teachers recruited to the RCS were new, requiring a range of resources to support them in their understanding of the curriculum content and their roles. The university funded a high-speed Internet connection to each office. Each RCS student was issued a laptop in a standard configuration that was loaded with the electronic resources that were available to urban students over the faculty computer network. Video-conference capability was established in the local hospital at RCS's cost. The university also funded housing for students and Internet connection from these homes. An RCS stu-

dent handbook was compiled, as was a comprehensive handbook for RCS medical coordinators, which included pedagogical support material for new teachers as well as an outline of the curriculum.

Although the RCS students were studying the same curriculum and taking the same final examinations as the urban cohort, their "program of learning" was different. RCS students did not move sequentially through the same discrete clinical specialty rotations as did their colleagues in the city hospitals. In addition, there was a considerable self-directed component to the learning style that was supported by the provision of the high-speed Internet access and a UWA-developed flexible tutorial system called "Flying Fish." Students enjoyed the excellence of teaching and learning opportunities in their rural sites and felt the longer rotation allowed them to become known to their teachers, who are then able to easily assess the type of contribution that is appropriate for their students to undertake. Students then became full participating members of the health care team, rather than observing learners. Students' emotional attachment to rural living comes from connecting to local people and spending time in their communities. The greater understanding of the dynamics of rural communities, and the opportunities for primary health care with those communities, will become one of the substantial legacies of the RCS training program (Denz-Penhey et al. 2005). Four years after graduation, 35 percent of the graduates had chosen general practice, and those students who had lived in a rural area were more likely to practice in a rural location, as were those who had been influenced to study medicine by a doctor (Ward, Kamien, and Lopez 2004).

UWA also offered a four-day rural placement to fourth-year students who were interested in a career in rural general practice. The program was titled Alternative Curricular Options in Rural Networks. Of the 103 students who participated, 81 percent expressed an interest in a rural career after the placement, whereas before this experience only 48 percent had been interested. Students also recorded a wide range of learning experiences, both clinical and procedural, and expressed positive attitudes toward the variety of experiences and the role of the rural GP. This program demonstrates that early exposure to rural general practice enhances students' interest in a potential rural practice career and provides them with a broad range of experiences (Talbot and Ward 2000).

3. At the University of Adelaide, the Rural Undergraduate Support and Coordination program has developed a rural week program for first- and

second-year students (Newbury et al. 2005). First-year students increased their knowledge of and interest in rural medicine and enjoyed their (limited) clinical interactions with patients. Second-year students appreciated the clinical experience and valued the welcome they received from doctors and practice staff. General practitioners valued contributing to student knowledge and skills and the opportunity to promote rural practice. Volunteer community members were enthusiastic about meeting the students, and their generosity had a significant impact on the students' ideas about rural lifestyle (Newbury et al. 2005).

4. At the University of Queensland School of Medicine, students in the third year could complete their educational requirements in urban Brisbane and through the rural clinical division in regional tours across the state. The rural third-year program replicates the urban one in terms of structure, curriculum, learning objectives, and assessments for each rotation, and all students take the same examination at the end of the fourth year. Almost all teaching in the rural division is delivered by local staff, with a significant infrastructure of offices, student accommodations, library resources, and information technology. For the 2002 cohort, there were no statistically significant differences in academic performance between rural and urban students. For the 2003 cohort, the only significant difference was a higher score for rural students in the end of the fourth-year clinical examination (Baumgart 2005; Carroll and Christakis 2004; Fischer et al. 2003; Garritty and El Emam 2006; Scott, Wilson, and Gowans 2005). For the 2004 cohort, rural students scored higher in the medicine rotation. The findings demonstrated that medical students learning in this rural setting suffer no academic disadvantage compared with students learning in the more traditional urban tertiary teaching hospital environment (Waters et al. 2006). The experiences of the medical schools in Australia present evidence that rural clinical settings provide an effective alternative to metropolitan teaching hospitals for clinical placement of medical students.

5. Similar to Australia, all medical schools in Canada provide rural training opportunities. At the University of Calgary, the family medicine clerkship is a four-week mandatory rotation in the final year of the three-year program. As a result of this rural educational experience, all students were more likely to do a rural locum. However, students from rural backgrounds were more likely to consider rural locums and rural practice, irrespective of participating in a rural educational experience. They seem

to be more open or willing to practice in rural locations (Woloschuk and Tarrant 2002).

6. Promising nontraditional clinical clerkships in the United States include those that emphasize interdisciplinary continuity of care training as well as those in ambulatory practice settings, with underserved populations or in remote and diverse learning environments (Schauer and Schieve 2006). At the University of North Dakota School of Medicine and Health Sciences, the Rural Opportunities in Medical Education (ROME) program was developed as an alternative clinical option for third-year medical students. Students in the ROME program are expected to meet all clerkship requirements for surgery and family medicine as well as to make significant progress in meeting the requirements of the internal medicine, pediatrics, and obstetrics-gynecology core clerkships. Two students are teamed in each rural community participating in ROME to provide peer support and enable team learning. Prerequisites for community participation in this program include the availability of at least three board-certified family physicians and one board-certified surgeon and the willingness of the hospital system to host and support teams of students each year. That support includes availability of a medical library and housing for students and their families. Students self-select to participate in ROME but must complete an application and approval process. During their seven months in a rural setting, students become involved as first-contact providers and rapidly become part of the health care team in those communities. Clinical encounters, including problems and/or procedures, are recorded on a PDA. Contact is maintained between the isolated rural students and other campus students via e-mail and interactive video-conferencing for lectures, conferences, and group meetings. Student test scores (MCAT, Step 1, NBME subject exams) were not significantly different from those of students who did not participate. However, students from ROME scored significantly higher on the internal medicine clinical preceptor assessments than did students from the traditional track (Schauer and Schieve 2006).

7. At the University of Iowa, third-year students completed the required family medicine clerkship with either a rural community-based, board-certified family medicine preceptor or with several family physician supervisors in a family medicine residency program. Students completing their rotation in the residency program received significantly less experience than students who spent their rotation time with a single rural preceptor.

Students rotating with rural preceptors received more experience in procedural skills (such as prostate exams, EKG interpretation, cryotherapy, skin laceration repair, and excisional biopsy) and female-specific skills (such as breast exams, menopause symptoms counseling, pelvic exams and Pap smears, and contraceptive counseling). Working one on one with a dedicated preceptor allows both the preceptor and the student to gain each other's trust and confidence, paving the way for increased student involvement with patients. Although preceptors reported that precepting increased their workload by about 51 minutes per day, resulting in fewer patients seen and loss of practice income, many of them found the experience of role modeling for the students intellectually stimulating and emotionally rewarding. Several preceptor teaching qualities were significant independent predictors of their students' total clinical skills: delegation of appropriate responsibilities, clear expectations, and providing the opportunity for students to practice procedures (Levy and Merchant 2005).

8. The Department of Family Medicine of East Tennessee State University offers students a four-week summer elective in rural areas of southern Appalachia. Students from 95 medical schools have participated in the Appalachian Preceptorship Program. The program combines an individual community-based preceptorship with an interactive group instructional block, emphasizes rural medicine, and provides students an understanding of the interface between culture and medicine in southern Appalachia. The group instructional block provides students a cultural, spiritual, and historical context for the delivery of primary care in Appalachia. A field trip to a local farm offers an opportunity to appreciate the uniqueness and substantial health risks associated with farming in the region as well as additional exposure to the values of rural multigenerational families. One of the greatest ongoing challenges is arranging housing for students in small, often poor, rural communities. In recruiting preceptors, faculty address this challenge up front and have offered rural office staff a small finder's fee to locate suitable housing for students. Students' evaluations have indicated that their commitment to family medicine and to rural medicine increased as a result of this preceptorship program. Those completing the program were more than three times as likely to practice in a rural community compared with the national average (Lang et al. 2005).

9. At the University of Nebraska Medical Center, the family medicine

rural preceptorship has long been the highest-rated required clinical rotation by students in the College of Medicine. Students value the preceptorship for several reasons. First, the exposure to an undifferentiated patient population allows medical students an opportunity to view disease processes of interest regardless of the student's specialty preference. Second, the preceptorship provides a "real world" taste of ambulatory primary care, a one-to-one student/preceptor ratio, and the chance to use and integrate previously acquired knowledge and skills to evaluate and treat common problems. Students in rural locations did not have statistically significant differences in their perceptions of either their clinical skills or comfort with basic diagnoses. Women improved more than men on technical skills, while men improved more on items related to women's health and psychosocial issues. This study demonstrated that clerkship coordinators can send students to rural areas with no degradation of educational quality as measured by students' perceptions of skill confidence. Proven educational equivalency, regardless of site rurality, may help medical schools and family medicine departments as they attempt to recruit and retain community physician preceptors to train medical students by expanding the pool of potential preceptors (Lacy, Paulman, and Hartman 2005).

10. The Rural Medical Education Program (RMED) of the State University of New York (SUNY) Upstate Medical University is a 36-week clinical experience in rural communities for medical students. A hallmark of the program, which began in 1989, is that most training occurs concurrently and longitudinally. In addition to clinical training, students visit community agencies and conduct community projects. Students also participate in monthly faculty site visits, during which they present cases to visiting faculty from SUNY Upstate's main campus, and in three communication skill sessions that include real or simulated patients with videotape review. Students live in apartments or houses provided by the local community. All of the hospital administrators were pleased with the RMED program and valued having RMED students. None of the administrators regretted participating because all felt that the benefits that accrued to their hospitals far outweighed any costs. The administrators cited the following specific benefits for their hospitals: (1) influencing students to practice in rural areas in the future; (2) retention of existing medical staff; (3) better care from physicians—participation in RMED was likely to help their medical staff remain up to date by wanting to stay current so they

would be seen as good teachers, and they would hear about new advances by attending conferences given by SUNY Upstate visiting faculty; (4) benefits to medical staff; (5) benefits to nursing staff; (6) good public relations; and (7) stimulus to improve the library. The administrators also believed RMED benefited students by providing comprehensive training, providing a greater involvement in patient care, teaching that health care in rural areas is as good as it is in urban areas, and educating about the administrative issues of running a small hospital. RMED students had significantly higher Step 2 scores than did non-RMED graduates. Approximately one-quarter of RMED graduates in clinical practice are located in communities of fewer than 50,000, nearly four times the proportion of SUNY Upstate graduates who have not participated in RMED. RMED has been similarly successful in placing physicians in rural New York state, with RMED graduates having more than five times the likelihood of rural practice as non-RMED graduates (Smucny et al. 2005).

11. The Rural Physician Associate Program (RPAP) at the University of Minnesota Medical School has 34 years' experience in training 1,097 medical students as independent distance learners in a community-based, continuity, primary care experience. The RPAP is a 36-week, community-based elective available annually to 40 third-year medical students. During the nine months, RPAP students experience the lifestyle of rural physicians by living, learning, and working in the community. Each student, along with his or her family, is sent to a different community. While in RPAP, participants evaluate and treat patients under supervision in the clinic, hospital, emergency room, and extended care facilities; assist in surgery and labor and delivery; consult with interdisciplinary health care professionals; serve as a resource to the community; and participate in educational activities such as a videotaped patient interview, formal case presentations, online rural medicine modules with online journal questions, online lectures, online interactive cases, and projects in evidence-based medicine and community health (Halaas 2005).

12. The Physician Shortage Area Program (PSAP) was established at Jefferson Medical College in 1974. The PSAP recruits and selectively admits medical school applicants who have grown up in a rural area and intend to practice family medicine in rural and underserved areas, especially in Pennsylvania. During medical school, PSAP students have family physician–faculty advisors, take their required third-year family medicine clerkship in a rural location, take their senior outpatient subinternship in

family medicine (usually at a rural preceptorship), and receive a small amount of additional financial aid (almost entirely in the form of loans). Upon completion of medical school, PSAP graduates are expected to complete a residency in family practice and to practice family medicine in rural and underserved areas, although no formal mechanism exists to ensure compliance. The PSAP program has made a substantial contribution to the supply of physicians practicing in rural and underserved areas and has had an extremely high rate of retention. Although the PSAP is a small program, averaging only fifteen graduates per year, it has had a disproportionate impact on the rural physician workforce. The PSAP graduates, who represent only one of every 100 Pennsylvania medical school graduates, account for one of every five family physicians practicing in rural Pennsylvania who graduated from these schools (Rabinowitz et al. 1999). PSAP graduates are the first to show long-term retention rates that are longer than the median duration, with more than two-thirds of PSAP graduates remaining in family medicine in the same rural area after eleven to sixteen years (Rabinowitz et al. 2005).

Graduate Medical Education

Most data support the fact that the postgraduate residency experience is important to the recruitment and retention of physicians in rural areas (Brooks et al. 2002). For example, 80 percent of Indian Health Service (IHS) physicians who teach felt that working with students and residents improves their job satisfaction (Brown and Birnbaum 2005). Eighty-four percent of the nineteen IHS clinical directors with teaching programs at their service units feel that a student/resident program is important to physician recruiting efforts (Brown and Birnbaum 2005). In general, these programs increased physician recruitment and retention, led to student standardized testing scores equivalent to their nonrural counterparts, and led to an increased sense of resident contribution.

At the graduate medical education level, rural training tracks (RTT) in family medicine residency programs have been developed to increase the rural provider supply by improving the education and training of medical students and residents in rural areas (Rabinowitz et al. 2005). One-two Rural Residency Track is an example of one successful program that contributes to the solution of the issues faced by physicians in rural areas. The program—residents complete the first year of training in an urban center and years two and three in a distant, rural community—offers comprehensive, ongoing training (Brooks et al. 2002). Thomas C. Rosenthal and colleagues have surveyed the thirteen RTT programs across the United States (1998). Seventy-six percent of the 99 graduates of these programs were practicing in rural areas, compared with 30 percent of all U.S. family practice graduates in 1996. In a small, cross-sectional follow-up study of graduates of the RTT programs between 1988 and 1997, 76 percent again were found to be practicing in rural locations, and 61 percent of these practiced in Health Professional Shortage Areas (Rosenthal, McGuigan, and Anderson 2000). Seventy percent were in their original practice sites, and, of those who had moved, 63 percent had gone from one rural location to another. Importantly, 72 percent of these respondents indicated their intentions to stay in their current locations indefinitely (Brooks et al. 2002; Rosenthal, McGuigan, and Anderson 2000).

1. The University of New Mexico (UNM) School of Medicine's Department of Family and Community Medicine has worked with its legislature and community partners to fashion a family medicine residency that addresses the health needs of rural New Mexicans. The success of New Mexico's family medicine residencies has been heavily dependent on this vision and commitment of the state legislature and community hospitals. Successful recruitment of family medicine graduates to New Mexico's rural communities contributed to their economic health. Residents and graduates have stabilized fragile health systems in crisis, adding new services in areas of critical need, and, through academic affiliation, have attracted other physicians to relocate there. Community hospitals have funded rural residencies, rural banks offer low interest loans to new recruits, and important manufacturing, tourist, and prison industries have decided to locate in New Mexico's rural communities (Pacheco et al. 2005). A greater percentage of graduates from the three rural family medicine residencies remained in the state and practiced in rural areas compared with graduates from the urban program (Pacheco et al. 2005).

The family medicine residency also created a state-subsidized locum tenens program, staffed primarily by family medicine residents from all four residency sites, thereby offering practice relief to rural practitioners (Derksen et al. 1996). Since the inception of the locum tenens program in 1994, 50 primary care resident graduates have chosen to practice in rural communities in which they provided locums coverage as residents (Derksen et al. 1996; Pacheco et al. 2005). The UNM family medicine residency graduates have made an important contribution to the rural education of UNM School of Medicine students through their role as volunteer faculty preceptors (Pacheco et al. 2005). The availability of this kind of role modeling creates a dynamic continuum that supports the foundation of community-based medical education.

2. In Canada, the location of postgraduate medical training is shifting from teaching hospitals in urban centers to community practice in rural and remote settings. Family medicine training programs in Ontario are a model of postgraduate training where training is comparable for trainees in urban family medicine programs and those in rural, community-based programs. Training in the rural sites takes place in community-based family physicians' offices and regional and rural hospitals, where family medicine residents are usually the only learners. As a model system, the Medical Council of Canada Qualifying Examination (MCCQE) Parts I and II performance by family medicine residents in remote training programs in northern Ontario, hundreds of kilometers from any medical school, were similar to the performance of residents in traditional urban training programs in southern Ontario. Similarly, there were no consistent, significant differences in the results of the College of Family Physicians of Canada certification examination between the two groups. Conducting postgraduate medical training entirely in a community setting is promoted as a way to better understand and meet that community's health care needs (McKendry et al. 2000).

3. Canada recognized that the practice skills and knowledge needed for specialist physicians in rural/regional practice settings were considerably different from the university hospitals where traditionally most, if not all, of the training for specialist physicians in Canada is given. This effort became known as the "Can MEDS 2000 Project," which was commissioned to examine Canadian health care needs and assess their implications for postgraduate specialty training programs. As a result, the University of Western Ontario Faculty of Medicine and Dentistry (now the Schulich School of Medicine) established the Multi-Specialty Community Training Network (MSCTN) in 1997. The program enhances the rural relevance of specialist education and provides specialty residents in anesthesia, general surgery, internal medicine, pediatrics, and psychiatry the opportunity to perform part of their training in rural and regional settings. MSCTN was the first program in Canada to fully adapt the new Can MEDS roles into learning objectives and evaluations. The evidence-based, com-

petency-based framework of Can MEDS provided a comprehensive tool to organize outcome-based curricula (Rourke and Frank 2005).

4. In 1988, the New South Wales (NSW) Department of Health in Australia developed the NSW Rural Resident Medical Officer Cadetship Program (Cadetship Program) to help overcome a junior doctor workforce shortage in rural hospitals. A second aim was to increase recruitment to the rural medical workforce on the basis that positive exposure to rural medicine increases the likelihood of choosing to practice in a rural location. The Cadetship Program offers bonded scholarships that provide financial support for residents of NSW during the final two years of earning their medical degree. In return, cadets are contracted to complete two of their first three postgraduate years in the NSW rural hospital network. Many cadets expressing an interest in rural medicine (particularly general practice) saw the cadetship as providing a rural focus for studies, a chance to develop the experience and skills necessary to work in rural health, a way to experience rural medicine and country life before committing to work there later, a way to develop networks and identify a mentor, and a greater chance to be accepted into a rural general practice training program. Those in general practice were much more likely to work in rural areas, and those practicing in rural areas were likely to be working within the same geographic region as the hospital where they completed rural service. Adequate preparation for rural practice during the early postgraduate years is particularly important because it is often during this period that decisions about practice location are made. The Cadetship Program is an effective link between medical school and rural practice (Dunbabin, McEwin, and Cameron 2006).

5. James Cook University School of Medicine, the first regionally based program in Australia, has developed a rural and remote training program. All final-year students undertake an eight-week rural internship, having previously completed twelve weeks of structured rural placements in the second and fourth years, and a core second-year subject—Rural, Remote, Indigenous and Tropical Health. Evaluation in the first year included student questionnaires, site visits, interviews, and follow-up teleconferences with instructors. Early evaluation suggests that the rural internship provides senior students with valuable experience in the health care team (Sen Gupta and Murray 2006).

6. The unequal and inequitable distribution of the medical workforce between rural and urban parts of Australia has been well documented.

The School of Medicine at the University of Queensland (UQ) evaluated the impact of its rural clinical division on the intern workforce in central and southern Queensland. The evaluation consisted of a time series analysis of first preferences for intern allocation among UQ graduates and sources of interns (UQ, interstate, and overseas) from 2001 to 2005, and comparison of trends between interns choosing the Rockhampton and Toowoomba rural sites (UQ student placements since 2003) and interns choosing Mackay (a hospital where the rural clinical division of the medical school has no presence and no placements). First preferences for Rockhampton increased from six in 2001 to ten in 2005, and for Toowoomba from five in 2002 to twelve in 2005, while for Mackay preferences were stable at two. At Rockhampton, among nonbonded UQ graduates the number of interns choosing to work there increased from zero in 2001 to six in 2005. For Toowoomba, numbers were seven and ten, respectively, while for Mackay there were zero (Wilkinson et al. 2004). Rural internships are a positive first step in addressing the recruitment and retention of the rural medical workforce.

Interdisciplinary Health Education

Often, the solution to increasing health care providers is not to rely on physicians and medical students alone but rather to focus on other members of the health care team: nurses, public health professionals, and allied health professionals. Several programs throughout the United States and Australia have established interdisciplinary, interprofessional practice and education programs to improve recruitment and retention of rural health care providers.

1. In 1996, a shortage of health care providers led West Virginia to create a statewide, community-based program with a required three-month rural experience for most state-sponsored health professions students. Initiated using funding from the W. K. Kellogg Foundation and expanded using state funds and Area Health Education Center (AHEC) support, the West Virginia Rural Health Education Partnerships program affects three institutions of higher learning, 50 counties, and 332 training sites. As part of their rural training, students spend 20 percent of their time in community service and interdisciplinary activities. A community-based rural curriculum was developed to orient trainees to future rural practice. Data indicate an association between trainees' perceived quality of the rural

experience and their increased interest in rural health, social responsibility, and confidence in becoming part of the community (Shannon et al. 2005).

2. The Center for Rochester's Health, a collaboration of the Monroe County (New York) Department of Public Health and the University of Rochester School of Medicine and Dentistry and School of Nursing, developed an innovative education program that gives interdisciplinary teams of students opportunities to partner with community agencies engaged in research-oriented health improvement initiatives. The goal is to teach students skills in applied health promotion and disease prevention. The center has supported an interdisciplinary team of faculty to develop education projects that link teams of students with community partners engaged in population health improvement initiatives. The center found that using a problem-based learning (PBL) approach gave students the skills to work independently with community partners in finding local solutions to community health problems. Curriculum designers must be flexible in creating an interprofessional education program to meet the varied needs of students from multiple disciplines (Andrus and Bennett 2006).

3. Two outstanding Australian programs demonstrate the challenges of rural interprofessional education, from designing curriculum to evaluation to care team relations. Most medical, nursing, and pharmacy students in the Faculty of Health Sciences at the University of Tasmania have some exposure to rural health during their training, either through rural placement, rural curriculum content, and/or membership of the undergraduate rural health club, RUSTICA. Rural curriculum content in all schools is developed and delivered by professionals with rural practice experience. In a survey of first- and final-year students in medicine, nursing, and pharmacy that explored their undergraduate experience of rural health, the factors rated most important in relation to career choice were those related directly to the realities of day-to-day professional practice—professional and peer support, work conditions, and variety of work. Approximately three-quarters of those entering undergraduate education in all three health professions felt themselves to be at least "somewhat informed" about rural practice, but only medical students felt better informed by the final year. The data suggest that the task facing those designing and delivering undergraduate rural programs may be not so much persuading them toward rural practice as not souring an already established interest. The ultimate

measure of the success of undergraduate interventions will be workplace changes over time. In the meantime, the faculty acknowledge a need for more research into interdisciplinary undergraduate experience of rural health to provide the data needed for the careful design of coursework, detailed planning of the placement experience, and long-term strategies to address those specific aspects of rural practice that are of most concern to those emerging health professionals (Orpin and Gabriel 2005).

4. The Rural Interprofessional Education Project (RIPE) is a part of the School of Rural Health at the University of Melbourne. This project consists of sending pairs or teams of students—from general practice, health promotion, nursing, pharmacy, physiotherapy, public health, and rural health—on two-week rural placements. Student teams volunteer to work in multidisciplinary pairs or teams to complete a community-based project (CBP) as well as to learn about primary and community-based health care and the ways in which health and other professionals interact in various work places. The nature of the CBP was decided through negotiation between students and preceptors, based on the salient value to the local community. Placement sites included multipurpose services, remote and other community health centers, small and large general practice clinics and centers, district hospitals, bush and district nursing services, and drug, alcohol, and mental health agencies. The RIPE project had the relative luxury of dedicated funding for a four-year pilot project and thus was able to develop a range of assessment and evaluation methods. The results suggest evidence of some significant educational gains as a result of this intervention. An assessment of the program revealed a pattern of student learning that found personal attitudes to be more important than technical "literacies" or accumulated knowledge (Stone 2006).

Conclusion

Scientific studies available to health educators and policy makers show there are predictable factors that influence recruitment and retention in rural areas. Policies for staffing rural areas with primary care physicians should aim at selecting the right students and giving them during their formal training the curriculum and experiences necessary for them to succeed in primary care in rural settings (Brooks et al. 2002). One of the most effective ways to attract rural health professionals is to train people from rural backgrounds in programs with a rural emphasis (Rosenblatt et al. 2006). In addition, both medical student and resident rural rotations were found to correlate with later rural practice (Brown and Birnbaum 2005).

As this chapter has discussed, medical schools can take the lead in increasing outreach to rural physicians and in providing intern experiences for medical students. The medical school can create networks and relationships that provide benefits to preceptors through infrastructure creation (Baker, Eley, and Lasserre 2005), monetary payments (Baldor et al. 2001; Carney et al. 2005; Levy and Merchant 2005), faculty development (Baker, Dalton, and Walker 2003; Bardella et al. 2005; Wilkes et al. 2006), curriculum (Brooks et al. 2002; Margolis, Davies, and Ypinazar 2005; Pugno et al. 2005), research support (Genuis 2006; Hueston et al. 2006; Pacheco et al. 2005; Zorzi et al. 2005), technology (Baumgart 2005; Carroll and Christakis 2004; Fischer et al. 2003; Garritty and El Emam 2006; Scott, Wilson, and Gowans 2005), and CME (Fordis et al. 2005). Rural physicians who act as preceptors rate student teaching as a valuable part of their professional lives (Brown and Birnbaum 2005). Medical students who take part in rural rotations at both the undergraduate and graduate levels report more patient contact (Worley, Esterman, and Prideaux 2004), better clinical skills (Waters et al. 2006) than their nonrural counterparts, and similar standardized test scores (Schauer and Schieve 2006). In addition, these students feel that they contribute more to the health care team (Sen Gupta and Murray 2006) and have a greater sense of social responsibility (Shannon et al. 2005). The preceptorship model and rotating away from the academic medical center provide valuable learning experiences and exposure to a large number of important primary care skills and procedures.

Challenges remain, such as how to increase student and preceptor interest in such programs. Isolation and socialization in rural settings remain a large challenge for the medical student on rural rotation and for the physician in rural practice (Adams et al. 2005). Curricula for rural medical education must be tailored to the unique circumstances of distance learning, lack of peer support, and lack of infrastructure (such as physical library access).

A major challenge for policy makers faced with a shortage of rural physicians is how to work cooperatively with medical schools to implement and continue these types of successful programs (Rabinowitz et al. 1999). For medical schools, becoming more accountable for public problems

such as the need for physicians in underserved areas could be an important way to justify new and continued public funding (Blumenthal, Campbell, and Weissman 1997). Except for a few model programs that preferen-
tially select students likely to enter rural or medically underserved areas
of practice, medical school admission committees may be less often pri-
oritizing among applicants whose characteristics are associated with the
selection of primary care careers, particularly family medicine (Pugno et
al. 2005). Program development is a long-term process, not only for the
students but also for the institution and the community (Andrus and Bennett 2006). CBME is part of a multifaceted solution to the health care challenges facing rural communities today.

REFERENCES

Aagaard, E., A. Teherani, and D. M. Irby. 2004. Effectiveness of the one-minute
    preceptor model for diagnosing the patient and the learner: Proof of concept.
    Academic Medicine 79 (1): 42–49.
Adams, M. E., J. Dollard, J. Hollins, and J. Petkov. 2005. Development of a question-
    naire measuring student attitudes to working and living in rural areas. *Rural
    and Remote Health* 5 (1): 327.
Andrus, N. C., and N. M. Bennett. 2006. Developing an interdisciplinary, commu-
    nity-based education program for health professions students: The Rochester
    experience. *Academic Medicine* 81 (4): 326–31.
Baker, P. G., L. Dalton, and J. Walker. 2003. Rural general practitioner preceptors—
    how can effective undergraduate teaching be supported or improved? *Rural and
    Remote Health* 3 (1): 107.
Baker, P. G., D. S. Eley, and K. E. Lasserre. 2005. Tradition and technology: Teach-
    ing rural medicine using an internet discussion board. *Rural and Remote Health*
    5 (4): 435.
Baldor, R. A., W. B. Brooks, M. E. Warfield, and K. O'Shea. 2001. A survey of pri-
    mary care physicians' perceptions and needs regarding the precepting of medi-
    cal students in their offices. *Medical Education* 35 (8): 789–95.
Bardella, I. J., J. Janosky, D. M. Elnicki, D. Ploof, and R. Kolarik. 2005. Observed
    versus reported precepting skills: Teaching behaviours in a community ambula-
    tory clerkship. *Medical Education* 39 (10): 1036–44.
Baumgart, D. C. 2005. Personal digital assistants in health care: Experienced clini-
    cians in the palm of your hand? *Lancet* 366 (9492): 1210–1022.
Blumenthal, D., E. G. Campbell, and J. S. Weissman. 1997. The social missions of
    academic health centers. *New England Journal of Medicine* 337 (21): 1550–53.
Bowen, J. L., and D. M. Irby. 2002. Assessing quality and costs of education in

the ambulatory setting: A review of the literature. *Academic Medicine* 77 (7): 621–80.

Brooks, R. G., M. Walsh, R. E. Mardon, M. Lewis, and A. Clawson. 2002. The roles of nature and nurture in the recruitment and retention of primary care physicians in rural areas: A review of the literature. *Academic Medicine* 77 (8): 790–98.

Brown, S. R., and B. Birnbaum. 2005. Student and resident education and rural practice in the Southwest Indian Health Service: A physician survey. *Family Medicine* 37 (10): 701–5.

Carney, P. A., G. Ogrinc, B. G. Harwood, J. S. Schiffman, and N. Cochran. 2005. The influence of teaching setting on medical students' clinical skills development: Is the academic medical center the "gold standard"? *Academic Medicine* 80 (12): 1153–58.

Carroll, A. E., and D. A. Christakis. 2004. Pediatricians' use of and attitudes about personal digital assistants. *Pediatrics* 113 (2): 238–42.

Cronin, A. J. 1937. *The citadel.* New York: Grosset & Dunlap.

Denz-Penhey, H., S. Shannon, C. J. Murdoch, and J. W. Newbury. 2005. Do benefits accrue from longer rotations for students in rural clinical schools? *Rural and Remote Health* 5 (2): 414.

Derksen, D. D., M. Hickey, P. Jagunich, D. Chavez, R. Diedrich, and A. Kaufman. 1996. New Mexico's academic model for providing practice relief for rural physicians. *Academic Medicine* 71 (7): 708–9.

DeWitt, D. E. 2006. Incorporating medical students into your practice. *Australian Family Physician* 35 (1–2): 24–26.

Dornan, T., S. Littlewood, S. A. Margolis, A. Scherpbier, J. Spencer, and V. Ypinazar. 2006. How can experience in clinical and community settings contribute to early medical education? A BEME systematic review. *Medical Teacher* 28 (1): 3–18.

Dunbabin, J. S., K. McEwin, and I. Cameron. 2006. Postgraduate medical placements in rural areas: Their impact on the rural medical workforce. *Rural and Remote Health* 6 (2): 481.

Eckstrom, E., L. Homer, and J. L. Bowen. 2006. Measuring outcomes of a one-minute preceptor faculty development workshop. *Journal of General Internal Medicine* 21 (5): 410–14.

Ellsbury, K. E., J. D. Carline, D. M. Irby, and F. T. Stritter. 1998. Influence of third-year clerkships on medical student specialty preferences. *Advances in Health Sciences Education* 3 (3): 177–86.

Fischer, S., T. E. Stewart, S. Mehta, R. Wax, and S. E. Lapinsky. 2003. Handheld computing in medicine. *Journal of the American Medical Informatics Association* 10 (2): 139–49.

Fordis, M., J. E. King, C. M. Ballantyne, P. H. Jones, K. H. Schneider, S. J. Spann, S. B. Greenberg, and A. J. Greisinger. 2005. Comparison of the instructional efficacy of internet-based CME with live interactive CME workshops: A randomized controlled trial. *Journal of the American Medical Association* 294 (9): 1043–51.

Garritty, C., and K. El Emam. 2006. Who's using PDAs? Estimates of PDA use by health care providers: A systematic review of surveys. *Journal of Medical Internet Research* 8 (2): e7.

Genuis, S. J. 2006. Diagnosis: Contemporary medical hubris; Rx: A tincture of humility. *Journal of Evaluation in Clinical Practice* 12 (1): 24–30.

Geyman, J. P., L. G. Hart, T. E. Norris, J. B. Coombs, and D. M. Lishner. 2000. Educating generalist physicians for rural practice: How are we doing? *Journal of Rural Health* 16 (1): 56–80.

Geyman, J. P., T. E. Norris, and L. G. Hart, eds. 2001. *Textbook of rural medicine.* New York: McGraw Hill.

Giri, B., and P. R. Shankar. 2006. Community-based learning in a time of conflict. *PLoS Medicine* 3 (2): e115.

Halaas, G. W. 2005. The Rural Physician Associate Program: New directions in education for competency. *Rural and Remote Health* 5 (4): 359.

Hertzler, A. E. 1938. *The Horse and Buggy Doctor.* New York: Harper.

Hueston, W. J., A. G. Mainous 3rd, B. D. Weiss, A. C. Macaulay, J. Hickner, and R. A. Sherwood. 2006. Protecting participants in family medicine research: A consensus statement on improving research integrity and participants' safety in educational research, community-based participatory research, and practice network research. *Family Medicine* 38 (2): 116–20.

Irby, D. M. 1994. What clinical teachers in medicine need to know. *Academic Medicine* 69 (5): 333–42.

Irby, D. M., and L. Wilkerson. 2003. Charles W. Dohner, PhD: An evaluator and mentor in medical education. *Advances in Health Sciences Education* 8 (1): 63–73.

Lacy, N. L., P. M. Paulman, and T. L. Hartman. 2005. The effect of preceptorship rurality on students' self-perceived clinical competency. *Family Medicine* 37 (6): 404–9.

Lang, F., K. P. Ferguson, B. Bennard, P. Zahorik, and C. Sliger. 2005. The Appalachian Preceptorship: Over two decades of an integrated clinical-classroom experience of rural medicine and Appalachian culture. *Academic Medicine* 80 (8): 717–23.

Leung, W. C. 2001. Differentiation and undergraduate medical education. *Medical Teacher* 23 (1): 88–89.

Levy, B. T., and M. L. Merchant. 2005. Factors associated with higher clinical skills experience of medical students on a family medicine preceptorship. *Family Medicine* 37 (5): 332–40.

Lewis, S. 1925. *Arrowsmith.* Repr., New York: Signet, 1998.

Maley, M. A., H. Denz-Penhey, V. Lockyer-Stevens, and J. C. Murdoch. 2006. Tuning medical education for rural-ready practice: Designing and resourcing optimally. *Medical Teacher* 28 (4): 345–50.

Margolis, S. A., L. M. Davies, and V. Ypinazar. 2005. Isolated rural general practice as the focus for teaching core clinical rotations to pre-registration medical students. *BioMed Central Medical Education* 5 (1): 22.

McKendry, R. J., N. Busing, D. W. Dauphinee, C. A. Brailovsky, and A. P. Boulais. 2000. Does the site of postgraduate family medicine training predict performance on summative examinations? A comparison of urban and remote programs. *Journal de l'Association Medicale Canadienne* 163 (6): 708–11.

National Health Service Corps. 2006. *Join Us.* U.S. Department of Health and Human Resources Bureau of Health Professionals. http://nhsc.bhpr.hrsa.gov/join_us/ (accessed November 15, 2006).

Newbury, J. W., S. Shannon, V. Ryan, and M. Whitrow. 2005. Development of 'rural week' for medical students: Impact and quality report. *Rural and Remote Health* 5 (3): 432.

Norris, T. E. 2005. The universal importance of the 'pipeline.' *Australian Journal of Rural Health* 13 (4): 203–4.

Orpin, P., and M. Gabriel. 2005. Recruiting undergraduates to rural practice: What the students can tell us. *Rural and Remote Health* 5 (4): 412.

Pacheco, M., D. Weiss, K. Vaillant, S. Bachofer, B. Garrett, W. H. Dodson 3rd, C. Urbina, B. Umland, D. Derksen, W. Heffron, and A. Kaufman. 2005. The impact on rural New Mexico of a family medicine residency. *Academic Medicine* 80 (8): 739–44.

Pugno, P. A., G. T. Schmittling, G. T. Fetter, Jr., and N. B. Kahn Jr. 2005. Results of the 2005 national resident matching program: Family medicine. *Family Medicine* 37 (8): 555–64.

Rabinowitz, H. K., J. J. Diamond, F. W. Markham, and C. E. Hazelwood. 1999. A program to increase the number of family physicians in rural and underserved areas: Impact after 22 years. *Journal of the American Medical Association* 281 (3): 255–60.

Rabinowitz, H. K., J. J. Diamond, F. W. Markham, and C. Rabinowitz. 2005. Long-term retention of graduates from a program to increase the supply of rural family physicians. *Academic Medicine* 80 (8): 728–32.

Rosenblatt, R. A., C. H. Andrilla, T. Curtin, and L. G. Hart. 2006. Shortages of medical personnel at community health centers: Implications for planned expansion. *Journal of the American Medical Association* 295 (9): 1042–49.

Rosenthal, T. C., M. H. McGuigan, and G. Anderson. 2000. Rural residency tracks in family practice: Graduate outcomes. *Family Medicine* 32 (3): 174–77.

Rosenthal, T. C., M. H. McGuigan, J. Osborne, D. M. Holden, and M. A. Parsons. 1998. One-two rural residency tracks in family practice: Are they getting the job done? *Family Medicine* 30 (2): 90–93.

Rourke, J., and J. R. Frank. 2005. Implementing the CanMEDSTM physician roles in rural specialist education: The Multi-Speciality Community Training Network. *Rural and Remote Health* 5 (4): 406.

Schauer, R. W., and D. Schieve. 2006. Performance of medical students in a non-traditional rural clinical program, 1998–99 through 2003–04. *Academic Medicine* 81 (7): 603–7.

Scott, I., C. Wilson, and M. Gowans. 2005. Are personal digital assistants an acceptable incentive for rural community-based preceptors? *Family Medicine* 37 (10): 727–33.

Sen Gupta, T., and R. B. Murray. 2006. Rural internship for final-year medical students. *Medical Journal of Australia* 185 (1): 54–55.

Shannon, C. K., H. Baker, J. Jackson, A. Roy, H. Heady, and E. Gunel. 2005. Evaluation of a required statewide interdisciplinary rural health education program: Student attitudes, career intents and perceived quality. *Rural and Remote Health* 5 (4): 405.

Short, L. M., Z. J. Surprenant, and J. M. Harris, Jr. 2006. A community-based trial of an online intimate partner violence CME program. *American Journal of Preventive Medicine* 30 (2): 181–85.

Smucny, J., P. Beatty, W. Grant, T. Dennison, and L. T. Wolff. 2005. An evaluation of the Rural Medical Education Program of the State University of New York Upstate Medical University, 1990–2003. *Academic Medicine* 80 (8): 733–38.

Smyth, P. E. 2003. Advanced practice nurses leading the way: A rural perspective introduction. *SCI Nursing* 20 (4): 269–71.

Stone, N. 2006. Evaluating interprofessional education: The tautological need for interdisciplinary approaches. *Journal of Interprofessional Care* 20 (3): 260–75.

Talbot, J., and A. Ward. 2000. Alternative Curricular Options in Rural Networks (ACORNS): Impact of early rural clinical exposure in the University of West Australia medical course. *Australian Journal of Rural Health* 8 (1): 17–21.

Thistlethwaite, J. E. 2006. Altruism can no longer support community-based training. *Medical Journal of Australia* 185 (1): 53–54.

Tolhurst, H. M., J. Adams, and S. M. Stewart. 2006. An exploration of when urban background medical students become interested in rural practice. *Rural and Remote Health* 6 (1): 452.

Turner, J. V. 2005. Awareness gained from rural experience: A student's perspective. *Australian Journal of Rural Health* 13 (4): 258.

U.S. Department of Health and Human Resources Bureau of Health Professionals. 2006. Area health education centers. http://bhpr.hrsa.gov/ahec (accessed November 15, 2006).

Walters, L. K., P. S. Worley, and B. V. Mugford. 2003. Parallel Rural Community Curriculum: Is it a transferable model? *Rural and Remote Health* 3 (3): 236.

Walters, L. S., P. S. Worley, D. Prideaux, H. Rolfe, and C. Keaney. 2005. The impact of medical students on rural general practitioner preceptors. *Rural and Remote Health* 5 (4): 403.

Ward, A. M., M. Kamien, and D. G. Lopez. 2004. Medical career choice and practice location: Early factors predicting course completion, career choice and practice location. *Medical Education* 38 (3): 239–48.

Waters, B., J. Hughes, K. Forbes, and D. Wilkinson. 2006. Comparative academic performance of medical students in rural and urban clinical settings. *Medical Education* 40 (2): 117–20.

Wilkes, M. S., J. R. Hoffman, R. Usatine, and S. Baillie. 2006. An innovative program to augment community preceptors' practice and teaching skills. *Academic Medicine* 81 (4): 332–41.

Wilkinson, D., J. Birks, L. Davies, S. Margolis, and P. Baker. 2004. Preliminary evidence from Queensland that rural clinical schools have a positive impact on rural intern choices. *Rural and Remote Health* 4 (4): 340.

Woloschuk, W., and M. Tarrant. 2002. Does a rural educational experience influence students' likelihood of rural practice? Impact of student background and gender. *Medical Education* 36 (3): 241–47.

Worley, P., A. Esterman, and D. Prideaux. 2004. Cohort study of examination performance of undergraduate medical students learning in community settings. *British Medical Journal* 328 (7433): 207–9.

Worley, P., D. Prideaux, R. Strasser, A. Magarey, and R. March. 2006. Empirical evidence for symbiotic medical education: A comparative analysis of community and tertiary-based programmes. *Medical Education* 40 (2): 109–16.

Worley, P., C. Silagy, D. Prideaux, D. Newble, and A. Jones. 2000. The parallel rural community curriculum: An integrated clinical curriculum based in rural general practice. *Medical Education* 34 (7): 558–65.

Worley, P., R. Strasser, and D. Prideaux. 2004. Can medical students learn specialist disciplines based in rural practice: Lessons from students' self reported experience and competence. *Rural and Remote Health* 4 (4): 338.

Ypinazar, V. A., and S. A. Margolis. 2006. Clinical simulators: Applications and implications for rural medical education. *Rural and Remote Health* 6 (2): 527.

Zorzi, A., J. Rourke, M. Kennard, M. Peterson, and K. Miller. 2005. Combined research and clinical learning make Rural Summer Studentship Program a successful model. *Rural and Remote Health* 5 (4): 40.

INDEX